Dedication

*To calm and settled hearts
waiting to surface from
beneath a blanketing
storm of fear*

ALSO BY DR WINFRIED SEDHOFF

A Balance of Self: A New Approach to Self Understanding, Lasting Happiness, and Self-Truth

The Fall and Rise of Women: How Women Can Change the World

The Friendship Key to Lasting Peace, United Communities, Stronger Relationships, Equality, and a Better Job!

TAMING FEAR

IN THE AGE OF COVID

DR WINFRIED SEDHOFF

Copyright © 2022 by Winfried Sedhoff

All rights reserved. No part of this publication may be reproduced, stored in a retrieval system or transmitted in any form or by any means, electronic, mechanical, photocopying, recording or otherwise, without the prior written permission of the copyright holder.

Paperback ISBN: 978-0-9946091-4-4
EBook ISBN: 978-0-9946091-9-9

Published by Senraan Publishing
Cover design and typesetting by G Sharp Design, LLC

First edition 2022

Disclaimer:
Many of the examples in this book represent experiences of real people. Names have been changed and identifying details omitted to help protect their anonymity. In several instances, I have created composites of patients to reflect similar experiences.

CONTENTS

Preface xix
Introduction 1

    A Bit About Fear 5
    Five Fears 15

PART 1 17
Fear Is a Charlatan!

CHAPTER 1   MEMORY BASICS FOR BEGINNERS 21
    Memory, Fear and Nature: How It Comes Together 23

CHAPTER 2   THE GREAT SIMULATOR 27
    The Worst Case 28
    What the Brain Needs for Fear to Go Away 32
    But I Can't Do Anything 35
    The Great Secret 37

CHAPTER 3   REDUCE THE BURDEN 39
    Stage 1. Box It: Compartmentalise 44
    A Worry Book 45
    Worry Time 46
    A Couple of Simple Rules 48
        1. Physically Separate Work and Home Life 48
        2. Do What You Say and Say What You Do 50

CHAPTER 4 THE POWER IN NOW ... 53
Stage 2. Use Mind-chill Skills ... 53
The Preparation ... 56
- 1. Set Aside 30 Minutes per Day ... 56
- 2. Choose a Quiet Place ... 56
- 3. Remove Distractions ... 56
- 4. Use a Comfortable Seat ... 57
- 5. Have Nothing Moving ... 57
- 6. Commit ... 57
- 7. Sit and Breathe ... 57

The Skill ... 58
- Mindfulness Skill 1. Zen-type Meditation ... 58
- Mindfulness Skill 2. Fish in a Stream ... 60
- Mindfulness Skill 3. The Off Switch ... 61
- Mindfulness Skill 4. Focus on the Breath ... 64
- Other mindfulness suggestions ... 68

Make Mind-chill Your Thing ... 69

CHAPTER 5 TAME THE BUSY ... 71
Stage 3. Shift From Busy to Happy, Manageable and Chilled ... 71
How to Slow Down and Still Feel OK ... 73
- Measure 1. An Activity Diary ... 73
- Measure 2. An Essentials List ... 74
- Measure 3. Do They Mesh? ... 75
- Measure 4. Take Time to Make Time ... 76

CHAPTER 6 THE CALM FOUND IN CERTAINTY 83
Stage 4. Find Peace in the Predictable 83
Methods to Create Structure and Routine 86
- Method 1. The White Board 86
- Method 2. Functional Habits 89
- Method 3. Know Your Job and Stick To It 91
- Method 4. Tradition 94

CHAPTER 7 CONNECTION REDEMPTION 97
Stage 5. Find Peace in Connection 97
Practical Steps to Tame Social Fears/Anxieties 102
- Step 1. A Strong Sense of Self 102
- Step 2. Know Our Friendship Needs 103
- Step 3. Build Your Tribe 108

CHAPTER 8 BEWARE THE NEWS! 115
Stage 6. Dial Down the Scary Stuff 115
Four Common Media Fears 118
- Fear of Missing Vital Updates 118
- Fear from Is It True? 119
- Fear from Factionalised News 120
- Fear to Gain Our Attention 121

Reduce the Fear Burden of News and Media 123
- Remember: Less is More 123
- Be Selective 123

Multisource	124
Connect with Community	124
Hold Media Accountable	125

CHAPTER 9   NATURE HELPS ... 129
Stage 7. Tap into Nature's Peace ... 129
It's Only Natural! ... 129
Nature Slows Us ... 132
Nature as a Balm for Status Anxiety ... 135

PART 2 ... 143
From Fear Monster to Friend

CHAPTER 10   FEARS BE GONE! ... 151
Stage 1: Preparations ... 153
Step 1. Find a Safe Place ... 153
- A Physically Safe Place ... 153
- A Mentally Safe Place ... 153

Step 2. Name It to Tame It ... 155
- Rules to Make Naming a Fear Easier and Honest ... 157

Step 3. Reality-check the Fairies and Unicorns ... 158

CHAPTER 11   FROM FEAR TO FRIEND ... 163
Stage 2: Hi! Time For a Chat! ... 163
Step 4. Have a Sit-down ... 164
Step 5. Have the Chat and Ask the Primary Question ... 165
- Will Acceptance Work? ... 167

Step 6. Call Fear's Bluff 168
   Direct Approach 169
   Indirect Approach 170

CHAPTER 12 MAGIC AND MIND TRICKS 179

Stage 3: Supplementary Skills 179

Step 7. Rehearse Success: Simulator Magic 179
   Why is practice critical? 182

Step 8. Combat Memory Shenanigans 184
   Building a Chilled Memory 186
   Dull Is Good 187
   Graduated Desensitisation 187

CHAPTER 13 ADDING JOY AND A TALE 191

Stage 3 continued 191

Step 9. Create a Joyous New Picture 191
   Joy Switch = Fear Dissolver 192

Step 10. Harry Potter It 196
   Paint, Draw or Sculpt It 197
   Write About It 198
   Play or Dance It 200

CHAPTER 14 MINI-WORKBOOK 203

Reminder: Fear Secrets 203

Ways to Reduce Our Fear Burden 204

Box It: Compartmentalise 204

Use Mind-chill Skills 204
Shift from Busy to Happy, Manageable and Chilled 204
Find Peace in the Predictable 205
Find Peace in Connection. 205
Dial Down the Scary Stuff 205
Tap into Nature's Peace 205
Importance of Reducing Our Fear Burden 205
10 Steps to Resolve Your Fear 206

Step 1. Find a Safe Place 206
Step 2. Name It to Tame It. 208
Step 3. Reality-check the Fairies and Unicorns 209
Step 4. Have a Sit-down 210
Step 5. Have the Chat and Ask the Primary Question. 211
Step 6. Call Fear's Bluff 213
  Direct Approach 214
  Indirect Approach 216
Step 7. Rehearse Success: Simulator Magic 218
Step 8. Combat Memory Shenanigans 219
  Graduated Desensitisation 219
Step 9. Create a Joyous New Picture 220
Step 10. Harry Potter It 222

CHAPTER 15 NO, IT'S NOT A TUMOUR! TAMING FEAR OF SEVERE ILLNESS 225

10 Steps to Resolving a Fear of Illness. 227

Step 1. Find a Safe Place 227

Step 2. Name It to Tame It................................... 227
Step 3. Reality-check the Fairies and Unicorns................. 230
Step 4. Have a Sit-down.. 231
Step 5. Have the Chat and Ask the Primary Question............. 231
    Acceptance... 232
Step 6. Call Fear's Bluff...................................... 233
    Direct Approach.. 233
    Indirect Approach.. 234
    Caution: Beware of Denial.................................. 235
Step 7. Rehearse Success: Simulator Magic...................... 236
Step 8. Combat Memory Shenanigans.............................. 237
Step 9. Create a Joyous New Picture............................ 239
Step 10. Harry Potter It....................................... 242

CHAPTER 16   I'M GOING TO DIE!.................... 245
10 Steps to Resolving Fear of Death........................ 247

Step 1. Find a Safe Place...................................... 247
Step 2. Name It to Tame It..................................... 248
Step 3. Reality-check the Fairies and Unicorns................. 248
    Fears of Losses from this Life............................. 249
    Fears of What Might Happen After We Die.................... 250
Step 4. Have a Sit-down.. 251
Step 5. Have the Chat and Ask the Primary Question............. 251
Step 6. Call Fear's Bluff...................................... 252
    Direct Approach.. 252
    Indirect Approach.. 253

Step 7. Rehearse Success: Simulator Magic ... 258
Step 8. Combat Memory Shenanigans ... 259
Step 9. Create a Joyous New Picture ... 260
    a. There Is Nothing After Death ... 260
    b. Our Consciousness Lives On ... 261
Step 10. Harry Potter It ... 262

CHAPTER 17   NO! NOT COVID! ... 265
10 Steps to Taming Covid-related Fears ... 268
Step 1. Find a Safe Place ... 268
Step 2. Name It to Tame It ... 268
    Fears about Personal and Family Health and Wellbeing ... 268
    Fears about Community and Spread ... 269
Step 3. Reality-check the Fairies and Unicorns ... 270
Step 4. Have a Sit-down ... 273
Step 5. Have the Chat and Ask the Primary Question ... 273
Step 6. Call Fear's Bluff ... 274
    Direct Approach ... 274
    Indirect Approach ... 274
Step 7. Rehearse Success: Simulator Magic ... 276
Step 8. Combat Memory Shenanigans ... 278
Step 9. Create a Joyous New Picture ... 279
Step 10. Harry Potter It ... 281

CHAPTER 18   I ONLY JUST SURVIVED! TAMING THE FEAR OF SEVERE TRAUMA AND PTSD ... 285
1. Demystifying the Ugly: I've Blown the Fusebox ... 288

Explaining the Symptoms 289

    What Is a Flashback? 289

    Why Do We Have Recurring Dreams of the Event? 289

    Why Do We Avoid Some Places and Events? 290

    Why Do We Emotionally Detach? 290

    Why the Aggression and the Anger? 291

    Why the Reckless Self-abuse? 292

    Why the Quickness to Blame Others? 293

Coping Strategies 293

Complex PTSD and Trauma 294

Using a Map: Want a Compass Anyone? 298

    Added Benefits of Fear Secrets 300

        PTSD 300

        Complex Trauma 308

CHAPTER 19   CHOICE AND HOPE 313

Appendix 1   The Balance of Self Model 319

The components explained 319

Personal Self 319

Family Self 320

Community Self 320

Land 320

Coexistence and the Balance of Components 321

Acknowledgements 323

PREFACE

Like most of us, I have known fear in many forms. I was ostracised in school, so fear of being different, not being accepted, and being made fun of was pretty standard. At home I was frightened of being physically punished for things I was accused of but didn't do. I was afraid the girl I liked in high school would reject me. She did, by the way. And I was terrified to fail a subject at university. Failing a subject meant failing a year and no more parental financial support. But none of these fears compared an ounce to the fear I faced one rainy Sydney day when I was in my mid-twenties.

It was an intense and desperate time in my life. Having graduated and finished my obligatory year of hospital internship, I was accepted into an advanced training scheme. A promising specialist medical career was before me. Still, I felt empty, profoundly sad, tormented. I had no sense of self, of emotional connection to anything. I was playing a role I felt others expected of me, and I couldn't keep it up any longer; I was living a painful lie. My solution was extreme.

Have you ever felt compelled to do something out there, irrational or desperate, knowing others would think it crazy or impossible, but you had to do it anyway? This was one of those moments.

I decided to resign from my training, knowing I would likely never again have the chance to be a specialist. Leaving was one of the scariest decisions of my life. But instinct and life experience compelled me to find the answers to the discontent inside me; it was that or end it all, and I did seriously consider the latter. So, I sat alone in a rental apartment, not working, living off savings from long hours of overtime. I spent most of my waking hours for months on end meditating and searching inside me, trying to discover an all knowing, a connection to all things, a sense of unquestionable truth – to find the genuine me, if it even existed. Intuition and my life journey had led me to believe that I would find a lasting, peaceful, comforting relief in finding this sense of profound connection.

It was not a smooth journey.

I cried. I blamed others for what I felt. I questioned and disregarded everything I thought I knew so I could look afresh. What if everything I'd learned was a lie?

My mind searched beyond me. Then there it was: a massive barrier of fear I knew I needed to pass.

In moments, the strength of the terror was beyond anything I had lived through or imagined. Every worst possible fear raged into my mind at once as though a wall of terrifying warriors had gathered to not let me pass. The images were staggering, of beasts, devils, threats to my life and soul. I grew up Catholic, and every fear associated with that religion rose to greet me – from eternal torment and damnation to forever losing my essence of being in a most horrible way.

What did I have to lose? My life? It soon became apparent there was far more at stake, and its terror was staring me in the face.

To make matters worse, I was set upon by the demon of doubt. I constantly wondered, what if I'm wrong? What if the truth is as I was taught? What if this is a waste of time? What if what I'm trying is impossible, as I knew many believed? Was I prepared to face the worst imaginable fear, beyond torture, abuse and brutality – losing my soul forever – just to see if I was right?

My heart raced, my body tingled. Sweat was flowing from every pore. I felt an enormous heat yet simultaneous cold consume my being as I sat on my bed with a pillow to my back – behind it, the sharp cold of a painted beige concrete wall. I focused all my will and concentration. The level of fear was immense. There was no going back. I had to get past this fear barrier. I wouldn't let myself be stopped.

Then the breakthrough.

A choice.

Fine, I told the fears, let's do this. Give me your best shot.

I called fear's bluff – all of them.

It worked.

As I let every fear consume me and take me wherever it wanted, I soon noticed them fade away. There was no substance. This was all threat. This was bark with no bite. Within moments all the fears dissolved and let me see beyond them, to see their origins, where they came from, and how they were created – what they really were.

With fear tamed, my mind opened. I wasn't afraid of what I might find. I was prepared to receive whatever there was. After all, my original goal was to see past fear's distortions.

What distortions?

Fear is a powerful emotion, and I had already learned that strong emotions cloud or distort our perceptions – what we can notice. Our feelings prevent us from seeing things as they are. They change what we see.

For example, when we are in the early throes of deep romantic love, we often fail to see the faults in our new beloved. We don't want anything to threaten the beautiful hope – the dream. It isn't until much later we begin to see parts of the real them. This is especially true once we have left them and moved on. Then we can look back and wonder, what was I thinking?

I needed to see past fear if I was to have any chance of finding what I was looking for. After all, we can't expect to see any sense of genuine truth if we are too scared to look at it and recognise it, can we?

Not much later – days or weeks, it's hard to recall – I found what I was looking for: the level of connection I had craved. It was a relief to know it was nothing like I expected it to be. That meant I was less likely to have just made all this up. Decades later, I would learn of others who had had similar experiences of deep connection to all. One description I especially related to came from a woman who recalled being aware beyond time in a way I could recognise immediately, though her experience came about when she clinically died and was revived. Her name is Anita Moorjani. More about her later.

Had I died? In a way I had, as was pointed out to me by a colleague and psychologist specialising in trauma. However, this wasn't a clinical death where the heart stops. The old me was gone, and so was my deep sorrow and torment – most of it.

Did this experience rid me of all my fears?

No.

The only fears that left me during this experience were those I faced at the time; all the others were still there. An accumulation of more than twenty-something years, all of them ready to be triggered and show up again at any time, as fears do. The difference now was that I had the tools to rewrite them and resolve them.

What do I mean by resolving a fear?

Resolving a fear doesn't mean suppressing it, ignoring it, hiding from it, fighting past it, doing things despite of it or calming ourselves until it passes. No, the skill I learned was to make them go away and never come back the same ever again by changing them on the inside, changing their nature. I learned to resolve them.

The experience of resolving the worst fear imaginable gave me confidence in dealing with other fears. After all, if I can overcome the worst that fear can throw at me, how bad can the others really be? Besides, now I know their secret: what the fears want from me.

I am still working to resolve my many fears to this day. However, I am nowhere near as scared and easily triggered as I used to be.

Am I expecting to rid my life of all fears?

No.

By exploring fear from the inside, I have learned that fear is there for practical reasons. To eliminate fear entirely is to be almost robotic and lose our humanity, the qualities we cherish. Fear, however, doesn't have to torment us, cage us, dominate our lives or prevent us from finding lasting happiness and comfort. It doesn't need to take away joy or keep us ignorant and scared. It doesn't have to trap us in a dark place as it can when fear rises to the level of a mental illness – quite the opposite. Instead, fear can help us realise the full extent of wondrous human experience and help us see beyond ourselves. Fear, I have learned over decades of resolving mine and assisting others in resolving theirs, can be a wonderful friend and ally. The key is to understand what fear wants from us and how to answer it. As we shall soon see, it doesn't want much.

Out of necessity, my life sent me on a path that just happened to teach me to intimately know and befriend fear, not as a goal unto itself but as a means to an end. Now, in the time of the global plague, life offers me an opportunity to share some of my fear-taming secrets and skills. The wall of terrifying warriors is no more. They don't need to be there for others either.

INTRODUCTION

Petra's voice on the other end of the line was a higher pitch than usual and lacked a strength of confidence I was accustomed to hearing from her. I had known Petra at our medical practice for many years. She had two children under ten, was healthy and happily married, and had been quite satisfied in her job as a primary school teacher. It was early into the pandemic, and most consults were via telehealth rather than face to face. Petra's prominent European accent was unmistakable, perhaps more robust, but she was still clearly understandable. Within moments of us starting the consult by phone, she began to plead and sound desperate. She then began to cry. 'Please, I can't go back to work. It's unsafe!'

The lockdowns in Queensland had been fast and brutal, but effective. New infections plummeted. Masks were mandated everywhere; even if you took a walk alone outside, you still had to wear a mask or else be fined. The police would kindly offer you a mask first if you happened to forget yours. Working from home became the norm, except for essential service workers. Now that the numbers were contained it seemed we finally had the virus under control: schools were allowed to reopen and accept students in the classrooms. Only teachers wore masks, not the students – back then children were considered to be at low risk of getting infected. Besides, we needed children to go to school, or their parents couldn't work. We particularly needed our emergency service workers on the job.

The media focused on deaths and worldwide case numbers. Many of us — myself included — would look at the Johns Hopkins website daily as if following some morbid sports statistics. Yep, they're up again. The deaths and infection numbers were especially going through the roof in the United States. But the USA was a first-world country with the best medical facilities in the world, wasn't it? What could it do to Australia if it could kill thousands in the USA? This new infection and the fear it brought with it was hard to escape. You'd have to be living alone and isolated on Mars not to feel the anxiety and tension. Clearly, Petra wasn't living on Mars.

Fear can present in many ways, from making us nervous, on edge, easily irritated and upset through to quick to get angry, aggressive. It can see us washing our hands twenty or more times a day and being too scared to leave our home. It can leave us constantly on the alert and worried something terrible is going to happen, yet for no apparent reason.

For Petra, the fear was physical. She was struggling to sleep and concentrate, she felt like vomiting at just the thought of going to work, and she would cry at the drop of a hat. But to not go back to face-to-face teaching meant risking losing the job she loved; work was insisting. What could she do?

'Can you write a letter saying I can't go back to work? I can't, I just can't ...'

'How long did you have in mind?' I asked.

Petra seemed to perk up. Finally, we came to an arrangement that let her feel safe — she had a legitimate medical condition; there was no problem there. She sounded so relieved.

*****

In late 2019, a new deadly illness most of us had never heard of raised its ugly head and would soon turn the world, and many of our lives, upside down. Within weeks of getting what seemed to be a regular cold, previously healthy people were suffocating, then dying. Whole nations initially denied it was a severe illness and claimed that it would be easily contained; it wasn't. We all soon heard about SARS-Cov-2, shortly known as Covid-19 (Coronavirus disease 2019) and then simply as Covid. One tiny virus soon saw thousands upon thousands of someone's mother, brother, sister, father, nanna, grandpa, cousin or close friend dying globally.

The effects of Covid were staggering.

Not only were there huge numbers of dead, but economies also began to collapse. Massive numbers of poorly paid citizens could not work, pay their bills or buy food. To make matters worse, there were sudden supply shortages and empty supermarket shelves. No one knew how long the shutdowns would last.

Some said we were panicking over nothing: this is just a flu virus, nothing more; we should all be 'free', not locked up and restricted. Some people still do. Social media went wild with disinformation, passing on unproven theories many wanted and needed to accept. We were all trying to deal with the new stress in our lives as best we could.

Covid has triggered fears in all of us. Petra's fears were a small but personally significant example of how Covid-related fears might present. Globally, according to *The Lancet* (8 October 2021) Covid has led to a staggering increase in the incidence of anxiety disorders: almost 25% higher than pre-Covid. It is uncertain whether

Covid-related anxieties will reduce any time soon while the disruption of the virus remains.

But Covid-related worries aren't our only concern. Over the last few years since Covid emerged, I have treated more people with fears unrelated to Covid than I have about the virus itself or its vaccine.

Life goes on.

Fear of being unable to pay the bills, losing a job, being alone, losing our partner, losing our home, losing custody of our children or something terrible happening to our family persist. So does fear of being hated by others and not fitting in, fear of past traumas that haunt us daily and prevent us from leaving our home. All these fears still bother us; they haven't gone away just because of a global pandemic. And when Covid finally passes as a major threat – and I have no doubt it will – our other fears will still be there.

To learn to tame only Covid-related fears in the age of Covid is not enough. We must learn to tame all fears. Besides, we can often tame our Covid-related anxieties by taming other fears too.

For example, Covid may have brought our fear of illness and death to our attention. As we shall see, both these fears can be debilitating in their own right. If we tame these two fears, then for many of us our Covid-related fear will also be resolved. We will learn how to tame fears related to illness and death later.

First, in the coming chapters we will begin taming non-Covid-related fears. Then we will see how the lessons we have learned can help us tame any remaining Covid-related anxieties.

Before we begin, let's learn a little bit more about fear and anxiety – what we are up against. This insight will help form the foundation for our approach.

A Bit About Fear

What is fear? How is fear different from anxiety? If fear or anxiety dominates my life, does that mean something is wrong with me?

Medicine is quick to reassure us that fear is a natural human experience, a normal part of being human. Medicine goes further to describe fear in terms of the 'fight or flight response'. Perhaps you've heard this expression before. In simple terms, this is our body giving us a racing heart, deeper breathing, sweaty palms, and twitchy muscles with increased strength and speed so we can either run away from or fight the savage beast – a typical fear response or reaction to something about to potentially harm us. Fear is there to help keep us alive and thrive, to make sure we don't miss out or lose what is essential for us as human beings. In short, to experience fear is a good thing and very normal.

But my fear is out of control; I can't do what I want to do. For instance, I feel agitated as if something horrible is about to happen. I can't leave the house to go shopping, meet friends or go to work. And if I do go to work, I can't concentrate; I'm on edge all the time. I can't relax enough to just talk to a person I'm attracted to, making relationships impossible. Fear is holding me back. Does that mean something is wrong with me?

No.

It might seem there is something seriously wrong or broken with us but, ultimately, it isn't true, no matter how severe the fear is – keeping us up at night, leaving us crying, agitated or curled up on our bed, unable to move. This raises an essential point:

> **No matter how out of control fear seems to be in our lives, this does not mean we are broken or defective.**

Neither are we weak or a lesser person.

This is worth emphasising. We are not broken or defective.

Why am I emphasising this point?

I bring it up early as a potent reminder as we move forward. I see many people who have been told that their extreme fear, known as anxiety, is a 'condition'; it is something they 'are' and must live with. I then see them given medicine and not taught any – or enough – skills to tame their fear. As a result, many get worse or insufficiently improve. We mustn't fall into this trap. Why?

Believing our anxiety or out-of-control fear is a 'condition' or part of some illness makes us think something is wrong with us and is out of our control; we disempower ourselves. We then hand fear the reins to become whatever monster it can be. That isn't how we tame fear; it is how we submit to it.

But I've been told by my doctor or therapist I have a mental illness, an anxiety disorder. Does that mean I don't?

Let us clarify. Medicine roughly classifies a mental disorder as a mental state that prevents us from functioning. There are different time frames of symptoms for us to be diagnosed with various mental illnesses. For example, to be diagnosed with generalised anxiety disorder (GAD) we must have anxiety symptoms (such as agitation, sleeplessness and a racing heart) on more days than not for at least six months. To be diagnosed with major depressive disorder (MDD) one of the criteria is to have depressive symptoms for most of the day and on most days for at least two weeks. Medical practitioners diagnose mental illness according to agreed sets of symptoms and time frames. It does not have a bunch of physical tests like when we diagnose diabetes or high blood pressure.

If our mental disorder revolves around fear, it is called an anxiety disorder. If we have no problems coping with fear, we don't have an anxiety disorder. Being diagnosed with a mental illness or anxiety disorder, no matter what type – and there are many – doesn't mean there is something physically wrong with us. Yes, we can feel more anxious if we have a physical condition, such as an overactive thyroid or have recently had a heart attack. Still, it can be unhelpful to believe our anxiety is caused by a heart attack or thyroid disease – a physical problem. It is more helpful to recognise that the heart attack and thyroid illness simply triggered many fears we now struggle with.

In terms of medicines available to treat anxiety, many medications can be helpful. But just because they help us doesn't mean it is because there is something physically wrong with us. Using that logic is like saying that we feel pain when someone stabs us in the leg because we don't have enough morphine in our system. The morphine can take some pain away. However, we feel the pain because our body is broken and isn't making enough morphine to stop the pain. That isn't true. There is nothing broken. The pain is a natural response to having three inches of steel jabbed in our leg. The pain isn't there because we are suffering from a morphine deficiency.

In short, if we have been diagnosed with a mental illness, it is a label, a description, not something physically wrong or deficient in us.

The first step to taming, mastering or controlling fear is recognising we are normal. Fear is simply behaving as we expect it to under the circumstances. How that is true will become apparent soon.

The next critical step in taking control of fear is to recognise that each of us has the inner power and strength to tame it – all of us, even those who have been most traumatised by it.

I remember many years ago seeing a documentary about a US Navy Submarine Commander in charge of a submarine carrying nuclear missiles. He was asked whether he ever got nervous or worried on a mission or about having to do the unthinkable and send missiles to kill millions, even though he knew that in the process he probably would lose everyone he knew. This is an understandable reason to be nervous: everyone dies on his boat if he fails; if he succeeds, he can wipe out nations. He said no, he doesn't get anxious or afraid, and I believed him.

Why did I believe him?

It isn't because of his military training; I'm sure it would have prepared him for his job. The reason I believed him was he said he had never known real fear in his life.

You see, this average-looking Caucasian guy had grown up in a quiet home, in a quiet middle-class suburb. He had comforting parents who taught him skills to keep himself calm and to be confident in himself his whole life. If something concerning showed up, he had been taught practical ways to deal with them and not let them overwhelm or bother him. As a result, there was no abuse, no fighting and no anxiety-invoking conflict going on around him in his younger years.

Lucky guy, huh?

I have often found the calmest people are average folk who just happened to have been taught or shown how to tame their fear – assuming they really are relaxed and not just hiding their terror. The reason people like you and I have struggled with anxiety is we weren't born into a home and place that felt safe and/or we weren't taught how to tame our fears like the sub commander was.

But you don't get it! You don't know how bad my fear is. There must be something seriously wrong with me for it to be this bad!

You are right; I don't know what fear feels like for you. I am not you. We are unique. Not surprisingly, no two people will experience anxiety in precisely the same way. How you experience anxiety will be different from the way it is experienced by your friends, neighbours or people you bump into in the street or see in the news, and different from the way I experience it. No one can tell you what fear is for you or how much it affects your life; only you can know that.

Having said that, how fear works and what it does – how it can affect us physically and mentally – we do have in common. We will see how in a moment. But, thanks to what we share about the fear experience, it gives us the confidence to know there are skills and understandings that can help all of us to better tame them.

Does that also mean all the skills we learn to tame fears will work the same for everyone?

No. That is where our uniqueness comes in. Some of us may find some fear-taming skills work better for us than others. Some of us may need to learn more intense methods and persist in taming fear more than the person next to us.

That is OK.

I remember a heart-warming story of an abused, terrified dog with barely any hair that would show its teeth whenever anyone came near. It was ready to bite anyone who came close. No one could be sure it could be saved; it was so vicious to everyone. But with consistent loving kindness and gentle caring, the dog came around after a few months. It welcomed a caring hand. It eventually allowed a kind and gentle pat. Now it was a happy family pet with a full coat of shiny, healthy looking fur, and could play without looking and behaving as if it was terrified for its life.

We each carry our own fear monster inside us, and in many of us it has been trained over many years like a vicious dog. Some monsters will need more kindness, compassion and caring than others. It isn't always easy, but persist enough, and even our worst fear monsters can be tamed.

That sounds well and good, but what if I'm too scared to look at my fears and what worries me? What do I do then?

First, we take a deep breath and realise that's OK too.

We will go slow.

We will begin by giving ourselves some space. We will do this by first understanding the nature of fear. This will allow us to keep anxiety at a comfortable distance between us and break the fear into smaller, manageable bits.

In the initial sections, you will learn the following:

- Why we fear the unknown. It's completely normal and OK, by the way.
- How our brain tries to predict the future all the time. We're being terrified by fantasies, and most of us haven't even realised it.
- The fantastic ability of our brain to rewrite fears. We can completely change fears when we know how to.
- Why fears can so quickly get out of control. To better manage our fears we need to be aware of how they can take over our lives.

Learning all this will help us better recognise, understand and reveal what can be regarded as fear's great secret. Moreover, this practical insight gives us new tools to master and tame fear.

What is the great secret that is the key to mastering fear?

Put simply, to resolve fear, our brain wants one of two things: either a plan or acceptance.

What a plan or acceptance is we will learn soon enough. Suffice to say, once we know how to develop practical communication with our fears, they are pretty happy to show us what we need, so they go away. Unfortunately, most of us haven't learned how to ask – to know the language fear speaks. A hint: fears don't use words.

Learn to communicate with fear, and we soon realise we have given it a bad rap. Fear often seems to terrorise and torment us, but that was never its intention. Ultimately, the fear monster just wants to walk with us and be our friend. Understanding the secrets of fear gives us the insight to embrace fear as a worthy ally.

At the end of this introduction, I ask you to write down some of your fears. This will give you a chance to ponder them before we work to resolve and finally tame them in the second part of the book. It will also help you see how some of fear's secrets apply to you personally.

Of course, if you prefer, you can write the list in a notebook. The same applies to later sections where I ask you to write down responses to other tasks I pose.

We will learn to tame what worries us most in the book's second part.

Why not deal with fears straight away, face them and get them out of the way early? Let's get into it!

Well, we wouldn't try to get someone to face and tame a major fear while they are running for their lives trying to get away from an angry wild bear, would we? The bear is chasing me! Now, what was that fear about work I was supposed to sort out? Ahh!

As we shall soon see, taming fear isn't just about resolving individual fears; it is also about reducing our fear burden. It is also about lowering stresses that add to our overall sense of worry or concern. How can we expect to master taming fear if we are so busy or scared all the time that we can't even find a minute's peace? It can't be done.

First, we chill. Then we tame.

Some of the skills we will learn so we can begin to tame fear by reducing our fear burden include:

- Ways to prevent work issues and worries getting in the way of our home or social life, and how to be more efficient in the process.
- Skills to calm the mind when we need to. Have you ever wanted to learn how to switch off your noisy, incessant mind?
- How to slow down from being too busy. Learn how to run life at sixty or seventy miles an hour, not one hundred and ten, or flat out – and be OK about it.
- How to calm our life by creating a framework of certainty. Simple skills can tame a chaotic, anxious life.
- Ways to find peace in connection. Social anxiety is common. Here we learn simple skills to reduce fears of being around others.
- Ways to prevent the media from scaring us out of our minds. Learning how to better manage the media is an essential fear-taming skill.

- How to stop worrying about keeping up with the Jones's and let nature soothe us as it was meant to. Learn how nature can calm and literally ground us when the world gets too much and our fears run rampant.

Once our fear burden is down, and we are more chilled, we will learn 10 gentle and straightforward steps to resolve fears such as those I would like you to write down at the end of this section.

In short, we will be learning how to apply the great secret.

Once we have explored and begun to master the 10 steps, we will apply them in a summarised form in Chapter 14, as a mini-workbook. If you still have any remaining fears, this section will resolve many, if not all, of them.

With the basic skills under our belt, we will learn how to apply them to two main fears:

- fear related to illness
- fear related to death.

Learning to apply the 10 steps in these two examples offers both practice and new approaches to further enhance our fear-taming abilities. Moreover, as mentioned earlier, learning to tame these fears helps resolve many anxieties that may be the foundation of fears related to Covid. After all, in any pandemic we are bound to face fears of getting terribly sick or dying before our time.

What about fears from trauma, such as those of post-traumatic stress disorder (PTSD)? Many of us are held captive by fears of abuses from our past. How do we tame them?

It is beyond the scope of a book of this type to comprehensively tame fears from complex traumas. However, what we can gain are a map and a compass, a direction to help us overcome our traumas and some steps to get there. Overcoming trauma-related fears can be frustrating and daunting. It is easy to feel stuck, and like we aren't making progress. However, sometimes a map and compass can be what we need. Therefore, the penultimate chapter has been devoted to recommendations on taming fears related to PTSD and complex trauma.

As we go along, we will learn strategies to overcome panic and other fears of no apparent cause.

As we have noted, Covid has triggered many fears. Many of us have become rightly afraid for the safety of our children and family, become frightened for our lives. In addition, we may be fearful of the vaccine or treatments, fearful of a new variant and new lockdowns and restrictions, scared we'll lose our job or our career will suffer, afraid we won't be able to pay our bills, and terrified to return to the social environment of work or uni after a prolonged time away. There can be many Covid-related fears that torment us. By the time you have reached this part of the book – Chapter 17 – and applied what you have learned, you will probably have already worked out how to tame most, if not all, these Covid-related fears. However, if you haven't tamed them, we will offer strategies to help.

Finally, once we have tamed many fears and understood their profound impact, we will learn a final critical reason why fear needs to be tamed: if we don't, the results can have a disturbing effect on our future.

The age of Covid is upon us. It is leaving many of us scared. Like Petra, we have been forced to face fears we hadn't concerned ourselves with in the past. We could let the fears overwhelm and dominate our lives. An alternative is to use the age of Covid as an opportunity. Fear has wanted to be our friend and ally for a long time. Why not give it a chance and finally get to know it intimately to enhance the quality of our lives?

What part do you want fear to play in your life?

Five Fears

Before we continue, I'd like you to write down five fears you would like to tame or eliminate. Start with what you are afraid of most. Don't try to guess what your fears are; you either have these fears or you do not.

Be honest.

It's OK; you don't have to reflect on them. Just list the fears then move on. We will reconsider them little bits at a time as we go along.

1. ....
   ....
2. ....
   ....
3. ....
   ....
4. ....
   ....
5. ....
   ....

PART 1
FEAR IS A CHARLATAN!

A friend I had successfully treated through counselling thought I might help Ellie with her concern. Ellie smiled as she introduced herself. She casually sat and crossed her jean-covered legs. Her hands were soon clasped in her lap. Tall and slim, Ellie's long blonde hair was tied up loosely with wisps occasionally falling near her right eye. Her voice sounded confident and precise. 'I think I suffer anxiety,' Ellie told me. You could have fooled me; she seemed calmer than a peach tree. We spoke some more.

Ellie shared that she worked in advertising part time and mostly from home, especially since Covid. However, the primary role that brought her a clear sense of pride was being mum to two young, seemingly well-behaved, healthy kids – a boy and a girl – each not much older than ten years. When I asked Ellie to tell me her greatest fear, tears began to well in her eyes. 'That after I've kissed them [the children] goodbye that something terrible will happen and I'll never see them again.' Yes, that will do it, I thought to myself. 'I just can't help it,' she continued. 'It gets worse on the weekends when Lee [her husband] takes them to the park. It's just down the road.' She wiped her tears. 'What's wrong with me? Why can't I stop these thoughts?' she asked as a plea for help. Ellie told me that her stress was starting to affect her work and sleep.

Quietly and sincerely, I validated this intelligent, rational woman's fears and concerns. She loved her children deeply; her caring and emotional connection to them did her credit. I reassured her that the fear/anxiety was something I was confident we could fix. She wasn't keen on taking medication and, having read my profile on the net, she knew I rarely prescribed it. I then introduced my approach, where I like to give people an overview of how fear works. Once we have a good understanding of the nature of fear, we can often see what will make it disappear.

I recommended two pieces of homework. First, walk for 20 minutes per day – no dog, husband or children allowed. She agreed. Second, write a list of every fear that comes to mind. We met again the following week.

*****

What I am about to share with you is similar to the explanation I would often share with patients such as Ellie.

I usually begin my next or first therapy session by taking more history and background. First, I listen to what the client is afraid of – often taken from their list of fears. It is good to clarify what they see as their worries or concerns as that helps me see how it has been affecting them. It also allows me to validate them. I learned that it is critical never to dismiss someone else's fear very early. Instead, we should respect that their fear is genuine, no matter how strange or unlikely it may seem to us. Then I would ask them what they know about fear or anxiety – what they may have heard or been taught. I find it useful, where possible, to build on what people already know.

Ellie had already heard of fear and the fight or flight response we noted above.

Earlier I explained some of the basics of how medicine sees fear. I see fear slightly differently.

The key to understanding fear, I find, is to understand some of the very basics of how our brain works – most importantly, the basics of how our brain creates and uses memories. As we shall soon see, fear and memories are intimately linked – understand one, and we can demystify the other.

CHAPTER 1

MEMORY BASICS FOR BEGINNERS

The brain can seem infinitely complex; after all, there are more cells in the brain than there are stars in our Milky Way galaxy. Thankfully, we can look past all that complicated stuff to understand fear. In the end, it is easier to see that the brain is ultimately very basic – in what it does and how it does it.

Suppose we walk into a room – I often use my office as an example. Instantly our brain is creating a representation of our whole experience of the room, of everything we see, feel, smell and hear – the half empty bookshelf behind me, the smooth laminated desk, the faint scent of the last patient's deodorant, the muffled sound of voices in the next room – and the emotions we are feeling at that time. Are we nervous, calm, joyous or sad? Every part of the experience of the room is laid down in our brain, just like every part of you reading this book is being laid down too.

How does the brain lay down this abundance of information? It does this through making nerve connections – masses of them.

Nerve cells in our brain don't just sit there; they actively make new connections with each other so they can send signals to one another and communicate. So, they are literally networking – though without the parties and the small talk.

Once the nerve connections are laid down, the brain can then reuse – access – them. So, if we were to leave this room and even glimpse back, that will trigger the same nerves to fire using the same connections we used last time we were in the room. You may know those connections as memories. Our brain creates memories using billions of nerve connections.

Whether or not we are aware of it, our amazing brains are laying down masses of memories all the time – all to be used again when our brain notices it is in a similar place or circumstance.

There aren't just reminders of what we saw, smelt or felt in our memories, but also what we were doing – more specifically, how fast and strong we were.

Why is a memory of speed and strength crucial?

It means we can get better at what we do.

For example, if we play the piano, we lay down what we call motor memories – memories of what we just did. So, the next time we sit at the piano, the brain will activate the same parts of the brain that allowed us to play last time. This allows us to get better by making new nerve connections representing what we did better. So, for example, if we need to play parts of the composition faster or slower than we previously did then our brain remembers our refinements – how we are more effective.

How about that? In effect, our brain is just one big refinement organ, always trying to make us more effective and efficient at what we do. No surprise there. If we want to survive, we need to waste as little energy as possible; constantly refining what we do allows us to do that.

It is a brilliant strategy. It is undoubtedly better than making completely new memories all the time because, unfortunately, that would take up way too much brainpower – a lot more brain cells and connections – and we'd need a much bigger brain and hat size. Better to modify the memories we already have – to refine.

How does this all relate to understanding fear?

The key is to recognise we were made to survive in the natural world.

Memory, Fear and Nature: How It Comes Together

Having memories that we can access and refine makes life so much easier, and safer.

If I don't have to learn to ride a bike each time I get on it, there is less chance of a broken arm or busted head.

Even more critical is creating memories of life-threatening experiences; otherwise, next time we do the same thing, we might not survive. OK, my mate was eaten by a lion because we were both too close to it. Maybe I should keep clear of lions – note to self. Memories are our body's way of saying I know what to do that will, first, keep me alive, then, second, help me get good at it. Memories are critical to our survival.

But we can't have memories for everything we are about to do. Some things will be completely new. That means there will be times we'll have no memory to use to ensure our safety. What do we do then?

Our brain and body have another brilliant strategy.

We need to realise our brains are made to survive in the natural world. So, when we come across something completely new in the natural world of trees, big rocks and dangerous wildlife, we have two main options:

a. act at the same rate and speed we do most other things

or

b. become stronger and faster and think and react more quickly.

Which of these two strategies will give us the best chance of surviving something utterly unexpected in the natural world: option a or option b?

Clearly, we're going to choose option b. It might be the first time we have seen a boulder rolling towards us or a tree branch breaking above our head and about to crush us. They are not the times to dawdle. Being faster, stronger and able to problem solve quickly is going to work a lot better than just moseying along at our usual pace – a lot less messy and deadly too.

What reaction of the body do we know of that makes us stronger and faster and able to think and react more quickly?

You guessed it: the fear response.

Simply put, nature has decided that when we encounter an unfamiliar circumstance, it is better to overreact and live than underreact and die. Besides, it's hard to learn anything if we are dead; at least if we are alive, we can learn from it.

We've all been through it. It could be the first day of a new job, meeting new friends, being on an unfamiliar road or just riding a bike for the first time. The next thing we know, we might feel a bit nervous, our heart starts to race, our palms sweat and we feel all jittery. We either get slightly nervous – a mild fear response – or downright terrified – full-on fear – or anything in between.

Think about it: how many of our fears are because we don't know what will happen and it is unfamiliar? Maybe more than we might initially think.

The main take-home point to remember here is that fear of the unfamiliar is normal. It is a vital survival strategy.

This is also an excellent time to remind ourselves that the natural fear of the unfamiliar is there to keep us alive and safe. Fear is on our side.

Then why do we worry about horrible things that might happen, like Ellie was worrying about something terrible happening to her children?

The answer lies in understanding that our brain doesn't just create memories of the past. It also creates memories of things that haven't happened yet – memories of the future.

CHAPTER 2

THE GREAT SIMULATOR

When Ellie eventually shared her greatest fear, I wondered if there had been some trigger – some experience – that had brought on her fear. The anxiety related to the children wasn't always there; it showed up only in the last few years. Had something happened to trigger the fear? For instance, had Ellie almost lost one of her children due to an accident or illness, or had someone she knew lost a child. If the latter, had she empathised with the sorrow, wondering how she'd cope if something similar happened to her? She recalled a friend almost losing to cancer a child of a similar age to her son and daughter. But now, Ellie wasn't just worried about losing them to illness. She had other scenarios running through her head of what terrible things might happen to her children, and they were intolerable.

In psychological jargon, it's called catastrophising, which means having an experience then imagining the worst may happen. *Oh, no, I've had this headache for three days; it must be a brain tumour! I just failed my first exam; see, I'll never amount to anything! Flying? Are you kidding? The plane's going to crash for sure!*

Our brain turns simple possibilities into complete disasters – worst-case scenarios – before they've happened, and often without any legitimate reason. In the case of Ellie, she had a good reason to imagine her children might get seriously ill, but her worst case wasn't about that.

We are all familiar with our brains creating worst-case scenarios. Our brain's ability to make the worst possibilities is entirely normal, as we shall soon see. This is the brain doing its job – as it is doing its job for Ellie, her worst case being she'd never see her children again. How we respond to our brain creating over-the-top worst cases is a different matter we will look at in a moment.

Look back at your list of fears. How many worries did you write down earlier that imagine the very worst and are still scaring the bejeebers out of you? A few? Most of them?

Understanding how the brain creates the worst-case scenario offers up its greatest secrets of all.

So, what are worst-case scenarios, and how does our brain make them?

The Worst Case

We now know our brain uses memories of the past to keep it safe. But how awesome would it be if our brain could create memories to avoid threats that we haven't experienced yet – like peering into the future to keep us out of trouble?

How great would it be, for instance, to know ahead of time about the car accident before we were in it or about the crane falling across the road as we walk underneath or the hold-up as we enter the store, and to know to stay away from work when some nut intends to take out a gun and start firing? Predicting the future could literally save our lives.

Nature also thinks predicting the future would be fantastic. That is why it also allows our brain to create memories of things that haven't happened yet – what neuroscientists know as memories of the future.

It's incredible; every day, running in the background, our brain creates memories of things that are yet to pass. That way, it knows what to do. It has memories to call on rather than having to work it out on the spot. In the heat of the moment, we might not have time to work out what will save us best. We might mess it up. But if we have at hand a quick response we have already run through – a memory to call upon – then we are more likely to do what saves us.

All of us are predicting the future all the time. Most of these predictions we aren't aware of. Many can be found in our dreams when we sleep, preparing us for the next day, week or month. Often the predictions that get our greatest attention are what we know as worst-case scenarios: predictions that something terrible will happen, like losing your children in the case of Ellie.

So, how does the brain predict the future? Are we all born clairvoyant and able to see what will be?

That would be great. Then we'd know the lotto numbers. But, then again, if we could all predict the numbers each week, there'd be no lotto or gambling, no one could make money from it. Where's the fun in that?

Instead of accessing the actual future, our brain creates predictions using what it already has: memories of what has already happened, and we have plenty of those.

When creating a memory of the future, all the brain has to do is make a few more connections that link together current memories. It jumbles them up then extrapolates on a few. And, next thing we know, it has a memory of something that hasn't happened yet.

Think of it as creating a purple elephant wearing goggles and flying like a hummingbird. Have you ever seen such an elephant? Me neither. But we do have a memory of what an elephant looks like. We also know what purple looks like, what goggles look like and what flying like a hummingbird is like – most of us would have seen images of one darting nimbly around a flower; they are swift. Now put all the parts together and, presto, our impossible, flying elephant – watch out, Dumbo!

Of course, what our brain is really doing is creating fantasies. It is a beautiful fantasy maker, a creator of the unreal. Every memory of the future ultimately isn't real. Does our brain know these predictions aren't accurate? Mostly, it doesn't. It assumes they are real and waits to see if they come true. If they come true, it holds onto the fantasy (the connections) to refine and use again in the future – to improve upon it.

Yes, we are getting scared by a worst-case fantasy. But, of course, all our future memories are fantasies. It just happens that some of them are accurate enough to be beneficial and help keep us alive.

Knowing that many of our fears are based on fantasies will be important when, shortly, we learn to tame many of our fears.

Another helpful and practical way to think about what our brain is doing is by creating memories of the future. The brain is simply running simulations, rehearsing for possible dangers. It is like pilots practising in flight simulators to prepare them for emergencies. By practising, they don't have to work it out under the pressure of a damaged plane and alarms blaring as it falls out of the sky. Better to know what to do beforehand, so we are less likely to make a fatal mistake. Better to have a tested simulation than not have one.

So, what is a worst-case scenario, really? It is both a fantasy and a simulation, depending on how you want to look at it. Both are accurate descriptions.

But my worst-case scenarios feel so real.

Of course, they seem real or we wouldn't take them seriously and prepare for them, would we?

*****

By now, some of you may have connected the dots and been shocked by all this. I know I was disturbed the first time I realised what our brain was doing. Learning how our brain reacts with fears to fantasies can take some getting used to.

It gets worse.

Look at your life and ask yourself how much of what you feel is based on what you think or imagine might happen, such as what your partner or children might do, what might happen at work, what you will do when you get bills in that you can't pay or what might happen on your next holiday? How much of what we feel every moment of our day is based on our brain's simulation?

Yes, our brain is living one gigantic simulation. Most of what we feel – including sadness, joy and fear – is according to what we fantasise might happen.

In other words, we are quite literally living in and reacting to our own dream world filled with fears of our own making that are mostly fiction mixed with a touch of reality.

It reminds me of the movie The Matrix – the original – where Morpheus, a dark and mysterious figure, informs the hero – Neo – he has been living in a dream world. In Neo's case, the dreams – electronic simulations – were created by machines trying to enslave humanity as a power source. In our case, we make our own dreams and simulations, and their story determines how we feel. We are all literally living in our own dream world – some of us feeling more trapped than others. As we shall soon see, we can use this knowledge about our brain dreaming to assist us in rewriting these simulations and, by doing so, change how we feel. By learning to tame fear, we will gain insight into steps to do it.

Don't like your dreams and how they make you feel?

We can change them!

*****

The good news is, by recognising that almost all our fears are just us reacting to our brain's simulations, we can now predict what it needs to settle down the fears and why.

What the Brain Needs for Fear to Go Away

Here's an important question. Can we be afraid – have any fear response – if our brain didn't consider what might happen, didn't peer into the future?

Think about it for a moment. Take your time. Consider all the things you are afraid of. What is your answer?

The obvious answer is no. When the fast car almost hits us, our fear has kicked in by our brain predicting the car will hit us. When we worry about losing our job, our brain is peering into the future. When Ellie was worried about never seeing her children again, her brain predicted the future.

Fear only happens when our brain runs simulations into the future. Some of these predictions may be in a split second from now, some may be hours, days, weeks or months away. But in every case, our brain is considering what might be.

What about fears we have from the past, such as those from traumas? They can also terrify us, but they look into our history, don't they?

Yes, but every memory is a prediction of the future. Memories have no use unless they can be used again. The terrible memories of our past that haven't left us are also our brain looking into the future. Only this time, it sees horrible things happening again. We will look at past traumas in greater detail later.

In short, our brain only makes us afraid when it considers what might be.

Knowing our brain can only make us afraid when it investigates the future is an essential and powerful insight.

Why is this insight essential to know and remember?

Two reasons. First, it tells us the safest – calmest – place to put our mind: in the present. We will learn some ways to do that soon. Second, it means when our brain makes us afraid, we know it is running a simulation of what will go wrong – what will threaten us somehow – or it has predicted the loss of something essential to us, such as a close relative, friend or partner.

We are afraid because the brain created a simulation that made us afraid. It saw outcomes into the future and didn't see payoffs. It saw loss instead. Losing our job, never seeing our children again or the person we love leaving us – these simulations aren't filled with much to look forward to.

So, how do we get rid of fear once and for all? What does our brain need for our fear to finally go away?

It needs to know we will be OK.

In other words, our brain wants us to show it a simulation - a memory of the future - that has us prepared and knowing what to do, and with a positive outcome.

We may know that positive simulation by another name: a plan. Our brain just wants a plan. And our brain will keep bothering us with the fear - we will continue to be nervous or afraid - until we give it that plan to answer the concerns it came up with.

Here is a typical example that makes more transparent how fear works.

Have you ever been late writing a report or assignment? The deadline is getting closer, and you start to get nervous. The time gets shorter still. You get more anxious, and more often. The fear builds and starts to get in the way of meeting friends or watching a movie. Soon the fear is shouting at you and won't leave you alone. Now there is so little time left to get the work done you panic. Fear is at the max!

This is what fear does. It gets more insistent. It keeps bothering us more and more, nagging us at the worst possible times.

Feeling afraid? Think of it as fear shouting at us,

WHERE'S MY PLAN?

WHERE'S MY PLAN?

WHERE'S MY PLAN?

And the brain will keep bringing up that feeling of fear until we give it what it wants.

In the case of being increasingly afraid as the deadline for the assignment or report gets closer, the plan is simple: commit to sitting down and getting it done.

But why does our brain use fear to prompt us to make plans? Why doesn't it just make them in the background – subconsciously – without all the drama? Our brain could just solve its problems, and we could just get on with it: no worries, no fuss.

Perhaps it creates this fear inside us so that we get help.

We are social beings – people who find safety among friends. Perhaps this is the brain's way of saying it's time to share my lousy simulation so others can help me sort it out. I can't find a suitable solution on my own. By bringing fear to our consciousness, we can share it and get the help we need. Have you noticed that often we feel better by having just shared our worries; a problem shared is a problem halved?

How many of your fears from the list at the beginning of the book are because you can't see things will be OK because you don't have a plan?

So, we will learn several ways to give the brain plans that help resolve our worst-case fears.

But what about fears for which no plan will make a difference, where there is nothing that we can do that will change the outcome? How do we resolve them? Ellie, for instance, can't do much from home to protect her children if they aren't there, and she can't be with them every minute of every day for the rest of their lives; that would be ridiculous.

Our brain has an obvious solution but one we rarely master. We know it as acceptance.

But I Can't Do Anything

Have you ever told yourself 'If it rains, it rains. There's nothing I can do about it' or 'If I don't get the job, at least I gave it my all'?

It is remarkable that the brain plans and prepares for the future to keep us alive and thriving. But there is no point in the brain forcing us to come up with many plans it knows won't work no matter what we do; that would be a waste of energy. And, as we know, the brain isn't one for wasting energy.

How does the brain stop prompting us with fear to search for and make plans that will never ultimately work?

We know this experience as acceptance.

Consider a typical example.

Are you afraid of flying? What is the worst-case scenario? The plane crashes, and you die? Is there anything you, as a passenger, can do about that?

No. You don't control how well the plane was made and maintained. You don't control the level of skill and experience of the pilots. You don't have a say in what the air traffic controllers recommend. The outcome of flying in that plane is out of your control – unless you are the pilot – so there is no point in coming up with plans to change what you have no control over. If you aren't afraid of flying, you have already practised the act of acceptance.

Have you ever been afraid of what might happen and then realised, truthfully in your heart, there is nothing you can do? How did that feel?

I often experience it as taking a deep sigh, and the feeling like a weight has been lifted from my shoulders. It is like the fear just disappears, evaporates.

When we honestly feel there is absolutely nothing that we can do to make a difference to what will happen our brain stops yelling at us with the feeling of fear demanding its plan. Then we begin to know peace.

My most gratifying learning experiences have come from observing those who suffer a terminal condition or are close to death. Once they stop trying to change the outcome and accept there is nothing more they can do, they fall into a state of deep calm and peace. Until that moment, they can be riddled with fear or terror. More about that later.

The point is, we can't fake acceptance. If we believe the slightest thing can be done that might change the outcome, our brain will keep the fear levels up until we give it its plan. Not giving up control – not accepting – is often a significant cause of us continuing to feel unnecessary fear.

How many people do you know who are on edge all the time and always have to control everything? How many of us struggle to practise acceptance?

* * * * *

The Great Secret

What is the great secret to resolving – taming – most fears and living calmer lives?

The secret is to create a plan or practise acceptance. This not only tames our fears; it can even tame our traumas. We will learn how in Chapter 18.

OK, if our fears are just our fantasies, why can't I just think them away logically? If I know they are stupid or ridiculous, why don't they just go away?

Some might go away, but many won't. Why? Because to change our simulations that trigger fear, we need to engage them with our emotions; rewriting the simulations can't be done with reason alone. We need an emotionally connected brain, not so much a rational one. We will learn how to connect emotionally with fears and resolve them soon.

* * * * *

Ellie and I explored her destructive negative simulations – her worst cases and their origins. We reworked her horror stories and worked on ways to better apply acceptance in her life. Initially, it was a struggle to rewire them. Still, within weeks her fear levels had settled right down; they were far more manageable. She said that knowing what her brain needed to calm the fears, why they were there, and what they wanted from her offered great relief. It has been years later, and she is still doing very well.

* * * * *

By now, many of you may want to go straight to the steps where we apply this secret revelation to make the remaining fears on our list go away. So, let's get rid of them now! But resolving individual fears is only one part of taming fear as a whole. There are many other ways we can use what we now know that tame fear overall, so our lives are less anxious and afraid. Many of these vital fear-mastering skills are those that reduce our overall fear burden. We will explore skills to reduce our fear burden next.

CHAPTER 3

REDUCE THE BURDEN

Kallie lived a hectic life long before she gave birth to her two children, who were still under ten years old. She had worked ultralong hours as a lawyer in private practice; working seventy-plus hours a week was typical. Massive study hours preceded that. Now she was an advisor for a senior member of the government and felt her life was the busiest it had ever been and greatly rewarding. Sure, she shared the burden with an understanding husband – he was a great support – but there was no sign of a reduced workload ahead. Kallie was feeling exhausted. However, what haunted her and disturbed her the most were powerful, ongoing feelings of regret.

What was she regretting?

Kallie was starting to look past the business side of life and noticing she wasn't being there for her children nearly enough. She was terrified she'd look back someday and be mortified that she'd missed the most precious years of their life. And you can't get those priceless moments back.

It wasn't like Kallie didn't have the insight to realise why she was doing it; she knew pretty well.

Kallie told me from the beginning she was being driven by fears of failure and not being good enough. She could trace these feelings to her childhood – needing to impress her father, a busy academic she craved attention from. She'd seen a therapist before. These fears of inadequacy were now pushing her to the point of sacrificing her own personal, social and motherly needs. Self-care wasn't on the radar. Time with friends was rare. One-on-one time with her loving husband was infrequent too. She was willingly sacrificing her health and wellbeing for work success. Suddenly, Covid struck, and she was forced to spend more time at home. Then it hit her; her children were missing out on her and vice versa. Now she was also being tormented by the fear of failure as a mother.

Of course, there were other fears in addition to those of regret and failure. Kallie was afraid to be late, especially on work tasks, scared to make a mistake or to let people down, and frightened that there weren't enough hours in the day, to name a few. Kallie shared that she hadn't had a proper holiday in several years. Her holidays were always with the family and inevitably jam-packed, with no time to truly relax. When I asked Kallie if she thought she might like some time off to help her recover from her noticeable burnout, her reply was quick: but work needs me!

Like Kallie, many of us are burdened with a mass of fears that rule many aspects of our lives. Some of our underlying fears we may be aware of; many we may not. The heightened level of fear becomes ever-present, normal, in the background. Often it isn't until something triggers us – like a pandemic – that we realise this level of fear isn't normal, and life doesn't have to be this way. Then, like Kallie, we begin to admit we have a problem – that life isn't how we want it to be.

Some of us may say a certain level of fear is a good thing in our life because it gives us enough stress to drive us to get things done. Fear of failure, for instance, was undoubtedly keeping Kallie motivated. So, yes, fear can be a great motivator and help sharpen our focus if channelled carefully. Left to get out of control, however, it can be detrimental to our health and wellbeing. Then it has gone too far.

Whether you choose to live on the edge with fear as your bedfellow pushing you that little bit harder is up to you. I prefer to tame as many fears in my life as I practically can — reduce my fear burden as much as possible. Once fear isn't holding the reins, often it can surprise us how satisfying and rewarding life can be. Even learning to lessen our burden of worry a little bit can work wonders; we often function better if we aren't too stressed.

Of course, as we mentioned earlier, the other benefit of reducing our fear burden is it makes it easier to tame our individual fears. How could Kallie hope to tame her many personal fears if she let herself be driven along at supersonic speeds? She couldn't. Mind you, she was making it clear she wasn't interested in taming them, for to do so would get in the way of more pressing matters — work satisfaction among them.

Whether your aim is to reduce your overall fear burden in life or to better manage the balance of fear in your life the following skills will be invaluable.

Before we begin reducing our burden of fear, I'd like you to try this exercise. Its aim is to help you see just how much fear lurks in the background. Then you can be in a much better position to decide if this is how afraid you'd like to feel.

Worry and nervousness are a form of fear. How much do you worry or get nervous in your day?

Tick the following statements you agree with.

- ☐ I get nervous I'll be late most days.
- ☐ I often worry I've forgotten or missed something.
- ☐ I'm afraid I'll let people down.
- ☐ I worry about paying the bills.
- ☐ I always feel nervous.
- ☐ I regularly worry about whether my family is safe or OK.
- ☐ I rush everywhere.
- ☐ I can't get concerns about work out of my head.
- ☐ I vomit out of nervousness as soon as I wake up.
- ☐ I worry about what others say about me.
- ☐ I worry I won't get enough likes on my posts on social media.
- ☐ I get anxious that someone might break into my home.
- ☐ I worry about my health.
- ☐ I worry about other people's health.
- ☐ I get nervous about meeting new people.
- ☐ I worry I'll have a crash every time I get into a car.
- ☐ I worry about what others think.
- ☐ Most days, I find I worry about where the world is headed.
- ☐ I regularly have concerns about the future and what it holds.
- ☐ I never seem to be able to be genuinely calm, to be able to slow down or find peace.

How many did you tick?

Is this what you want: to live a life controlled by so many fears? No?

There are practical steps to tame them. We can start with work.

*****

A significant impact that Covid had on us was how we work. To help control the spread and reduce deaths, people were ordered to stay home and only go out if essential. Working from home became a thing. Who would have thought? We have been so used to working around colleagues in offices that suddenly working from home alone was a shock. Post-lockdown many of us continue to work from home for at least part of our working week.

Doing our job from home comes with many challenges aside from the lack of connection we crave. Many of us face the trial of not letting work take over our minds during every working – even sleeping – moment.

We may have struggled to keep thoughts of work and not constantly looking at our phone emails from interfering with our social and family life before Covid. Now Covid has made matters worse. Now work is within arm's reach the moment we wake up!

But our brain needs a break. Our families deserve our attention. Our social life requires us to be present; otherwise, we will lose even more connections, feel lonelier, and soon be burnt out.

Worse, not managing work and social life separately makes us less efficient. So, our work takes longer, and the quality can suffer.

Not keeping work and the rest of life separate means an unnecessary increase in stress. It can be a significant source of anxiety. That means a considerable fear burden we don't need.

Thankfully, there is a practical and straightforward fix. There are simple steps that can be taken to reduce our overall fear burden. We look at the first step - or stage - below. In later chapters we look at the remaining stages.

Stage 1. Box It: Compartmentalise

Max came in stressed about work long before the pressures of Covid and lockdowns were on his agenda. Running his own business from home, he was always close to emails and access to his computer. His phone was always a touch away; it was like never really leaving work. He couldn't get a break; work was affecting his sleep, relationship and social life. What social life? There wasn't time; he had his own business to run. It was like the dripping tap torture where you lay down, and a single drop of water drips onto your forehead every few seconds and never stops. Even the strongest of us can't expect to tolerate the constant, unrelenting drip without going crazy.

The key to fixing Max's problem is a simple strategy we can all learn: compartmentalise.

What do we mean by compartmentalising?

Think of compartmentalising as putting different parts of life into boxes with solid walls and a lid. None of the contents of one box mixes with the other; we keep them separate. Max's work is in one box, and the rest of his life – social and personal – is in another.

Max applied the following steps to the letter; he was keen to make it work. His results were impressive.

How do we compartmentalise our work and life?

All we need are:

- a worry book
- worry time
- a couple of simple rules.

A Worry Book

A worry book is a small pad with a pen or pencil you carry at work and home.

The worry book is there to write down what we might forget that needs our attention.

How is it helpful to write what we might forget?

Fear is one of the brain's ways of getting our attention. You may recall one of the secrets of fear was our brain would use fear to shout to us, WHERE'S MY PLAN? It's doing the same here, bringing up something important it knows needs our attention. And it will keep doing it – often at the worst or most inconvenient times – until we deal with it.

For example, you might be working on a project when you remember that you need to sort out the details of Ken's account and give him a call. We worry about Ken and his account. We mustn't forget. The thought won't leave us. We worry more. But, darn it, we must give in and call Ken now. Then we remember about Sabina's account, then Tom's, then Helena's. Distraction after distraction, fear after fear. Then, before we know it, we are behind in our other work, and the day gets out of control. The next thing we know, we are working out of regular work hours to catch up, and work takes over our life.

Sound familiar?

This is where the worry book becomes our saviour.

In the case of Ken, we would write down in our worry book, 'Call Ken!' Then, if there were other things that we thought we might forget, we write them down too. Then we get on with what we were doing.

Similarly, if we are at home – not at work – and work-related ideas or tasks come to mind, we write them down too. Then we leave them alone – don't think about them.

What makes the worry book work is knowing we will look at it, that the task will be dealt with. Then the brain is prepared to let it go. This is where the next step becomes essential; setting aside worry time.

* * * *

> ## CRITICAL POINT
>
> The worry book will only work if our brain is sure we will look at it regularly. If it isn't sure when we'll look at it again, it will go back to its old ways of annoying us with inconvenient fears at the worst possible times, and we are back where we started.

Worry Time

We all need worry time, time to specifically deal with our concerns or worries. Worry time is a must.

Why is worry time so critical?

If we have a good time to look at and sort out our fears, concerns and worries, we won't have so many piled up. We will be less triggered and distracted by fears as we have fewer to bother us.

As we have seen, our brain often needs our conscious help and attention to deal with fears. Hence, it will bring them to our consciousness rather than sorting them in the background. If we don't give our brain the necessary time to sort out the concern – give it a plan or acceptance – the fear will often hang around and show up at a most inconvenient time. So, we either sort out our worries at a time that suits us or our brain will find a time to worry who knows when, like during a nice dinner outing or in the middle of a job interview or critical task.

Worry time is most potent when used with the worry book.

Try this. Suppose it is a regular workday. We set three times aside in our day as worry time. For example:

- half an hour before work
- half an hour at or before lunch
- half to 1 hour after work, before we go home.

We look at our worry book and work out what worry needs to be sorted in those times.

Consider the following examples:

- Before work, we look in the worry book to see what we have written at home, between work hours, and the previous day or weekend. Then we either take care of each concern there and then, if we can, or have a plan for addressing the concerns during the day (such as writing it in a diary or list of daily activities). If the latter, we need to know we will follow the plan.
- Before lunch, we look at any issues we wrote down in the morning or new tasks we think are urgent and sort them out either within this half hour or plan for them to be sorted later in the day or week, again using a list.
- After work, we do a debrief of the day. We go over everything we did in the day, work out what needs to be done tomorrow and make sure nothing needs to be done that can't wait until the morning. Then we go home to our family, or meet up

with friends, or just relax and recover. We can rest assured our worry will be dealt with as we've made the time and/or the plan. We can leave the worries behind until then.

We should also keep our worry book handy on weekends. Then, if a work concern, task or inspiration shows up we just whip out our worry book, make a note, then put it aside to be looked at during our first worry time session the next workday. We don't mull over any work problems now; we don't let them take up our non-work time. Instead, we remain present with the people and places around us to enjoy other precious aspects of life.

Can we set aside worry time for weekends?

Sure, but not to focus on sorting problems from work; work stays at work.

We all need a break from work, no matter how fulfilling or thrilling it may be. This is true even of the highly driven Kallies of the world. Compartmentalising ensures we get the healthy balance we need. At the same time, it reduces our worries – tames many of our day-to-day fears – thus reducing our fear burden.

To compartmentalise well, we also need a couple of other rules.

A Couple of Simple Rules

1. Physically Separate Work and Home Life

Keep work and home life as separate as you physically can. Otherwise, work stuff will start niggling its way into your home and social life. Suppose you occasionally look at your emails at the kitchen table; for instance, the next time you eat. In that case, you are likely to start thinking about work and your emails; I'll only take a quick looksie. Sure, you will. We can keep work and home life separate in the following ways:

- First, in your home make a distinct area that is just for work. Do not work in common areas where the family meets, such as the kitchen table. A small foldaway chair and table set up in an unused corner might be the answer if space is at a premium.
- Second, keep strict work hours. Do not go back to work at the end of your work hours, especially not to check emails. Use your worry book instead. If you need extra time to sort things out the next day, then get to work early.
- Third, keep a separate work phone. At the end of the workday, everyone from work (including clients) must know you are not available. Your private phone is for everything that isn't work. Unless the office is burning down or there is an imminent nuclear attack, they never use your private number.
- Fourth, never take work on holidays. A holiday is to get our energy back, so we enjoy ourselves and are more effective when we return to work. The more we think about, or do, work on holidays, the less of us we offer when we get back. We won't be as refreshed, and our family won't be too happy we weren't there for them either. Where's daddy? Where's mummy? Where's my husband or wife? I miss them.
- Fifth, never over-commit. If you say you will do something you know you can't deliver on you will worry yourself the whole time about how you will do it, and no worry book will save you.

Max was quick to admit he'd sneak a peek at his emails after dinner. He'd often find he'd think about work when at home talking to his wife. He noticed he wasn't very present, even for the kids; his mind was often still at work.

2. Do What You Say and Say What You Do

Do what you say follows on from never over-commit. If you say that you will do something, make sure it gets done. This gives our brain certainty. As we briefly noticed earlier, giving the brain certainty is a great way to reduce fears in adults and children. We will also give ourselves a reputation for reliability by doing what we say. Anyone in business knows how important reputation and dependability are in a successful business.

Say what you do means don't lie. So, for example, don't say you will do something you know you won't do, and don't tell others that you did what you know you didn't: that is a lie.

Lies to fears are like catnip to cats: they feed on it and get high. When we lie, we worry about being found out and keeping our stories straight. This gives us too many unnecessary reasons to worry. Lies, obviously, aren't good for our business and personal reputation either; they often come back to bite us.

What if I'm not a list person? You mentioned using the worry book to write down a task on a to-do list or daily diary. Do I really need a daily diary?

To be honest, I'm not a list person either as I don't like the idea of having my day dictated to me; I don't like feeling too trapped or restricted. Thankfully, my days are organised enough and not too busy to need a detailed list, except for my list of patients for the day and other 'homework' I need to do before going home. Having the luxury of having most of my day organised for me wasn't always the case.

When I was an intern during my doctor training in a teaching hospital I carried a large notepad with me everywhere, especially in the mornings on ward rounds with the specialists. The notepad was the equivalent of my worry book, and the lists I made on it were my saviour. The list offered reassurance that all the tasks I was given would get done, and I wouldn't have to worry about any I might have forgotten. Better still, any jobs I couldn't finish or stay back for I could hand over to colleagues knowing they wouldn't be on my mind all night; I could switch off from the job. But, of course, when you are in a stressful occupation, such as a junior doctor, you need to switch off, or you are sure to burn out or break. So, I needed to use my own lists to organise myself. It worked.

If our days are filled with many jobs or activities we know we mustn't forget, then a daytime diary or list of tasks is a blessing. Instead of restricting us, the list frees us. It frees our time by making us more efficient – not going from task to task or being distracted – and frees us from a whole bunch of fears we don't need.

* * * * *

Max applied the suggestions we just described. He created a separate workspace at home, bought a work-only phone and kept a worry book on his person most waking hours.

Within two weeks, he came back looking like a weight had been lifted from his shoulders. His business improved, and his partner was happier too.

* * * * *

I have shared this simple method with many people struggling to work from home in a productive, less personally destructive way both before and since Covid. Often it is the only strategy they feel they need for now.

Of course, the same principles of compartmentalising apply to every aspect of life. The more we can be present and not worry about what we might forget, the less fear will keep popping up unexpectedly to ruin our day. Soon we will look at how to use structure and routines to help us reduce anxiety even more.

No matter who we are, we should all set aside worry time.

Compartmentalising is a powerful fear-taming strategy we can all learn to master.

*****

Another challenge that Covid can highlight is our non-stop busy mind. Being alone at home means being alone with our thoughts. There are only so many movies or TV series we can stream, only so many books or magazines we can read. Then there they are: our thoughts are taking control. To have an uncontrolled, busy mind is stress unto itself. It is a significant fear burden. But, it is also a challenge we can meet and master by simply learning a few skills. We will learn some of these skills in the following chapter.

CHAPTER 4

THE POWER IN NOW

Stage 2. Use Mind-chill Skills

'Can you make it stop? I can't get it to stop.' Stan seemed agitated, distressed. A slim chap dressed in dirty work trousers, shirt and heavy laced boots with a zipper up the inside; he'd just come from work. Stan was in his mid-twenties and generally healthy. Stan was convinced he was going crazy – 'Am I crazy, Doc?' His noisy, distracting mind riddled with images of horrible scenarios were getting in the way of his work. His boss was complaining that Stan, who had just finished his apprenticeship, wasn't focusing on the task at hand – and on a building site that can be dangerous. Get help, he was told. Now here he was asking if he could find a way to shut his mind off, give his mind a break.

I have had numerous people like Stan from all walks of life, from carpenters to school and university students, business executives, lawyers. They all ask how do I switch off my mind? Is there a switch? Struggling to control our thoughts is common. Learning to quieten our mind – almost entirely when needed – is an essential and practical skill all of us can and should know.

Many mind-calming techniques help reduce stress. They offer peace of mind and reduce our fear/anxiety burden. They can often be found under the heading of 'mindfulness'.

Mindfulness is a powerful tool to tame fear. Search the word mindfulness on the net, and you can find many definitions. Essentially, mindfulness is a state of being present in the now without judgement – just being here and noticing.

How does mindfulness help us tame fear?

Mindfulness taps into a secret about fear we have just learned: the brain can only be afraid if it considers the future.

As we have seen, worrying about what might happen to our children or whether we will lose our job or catch Covid are all examples of our brain checking out the possible future and making us afraid. So, look again if you aren't convinced: is there any time you feel fear where your mind isn't considering what might happen next?

As we noted, even past fears are our brain considering whether what happened in the past might happen again. So, they want to prepare us; our brain is still considering our future.

All fears live in the future, even if it is a microsecond from now.

The now is a potent and refreshing place we should all learn to visit, especially if we seek to reduce the burden of fear and learn to tame it.

* * * * *

This chapter will teach us four ways to bring the mind into the present through mindfulness or mindful meditations. We will mention other ways to engage in mindfulness at the end of the chapter. I'm not here to say one form of mindfulness is better than another. Instead, I will share the four I teach and have used, or developed, personally. The third is the closest you will find to flicking a switch to stop our constant pesky and intrusive thoughts like Stan was trying to do.

Meditation? Sounds weird, especially if you've never tried it before.

Don't let the term meditation put you off if you aren't familiar with it. Meditation is simply a way to change our state of mind, so we see or notice things differently.

We are about to apply simple mind skills. There is nothing supernatural or unusual about them. They are perfectly natural skills to learn, just as natural as learning to walk or run.

Like all worthwhile skills, they need some practice. After all, we can't expect to play brilliant classical guitar immediately after picking up the instrument for the first time. We will talk more about how often we should practice in a moment.

We will break down learning the meditations into two parts:

- the preparation
- the skill.

The preparation is just to set up the place to meditate. The skill is the actual practice: the meditation itself. Both the preparation and the skill are important.

The Preparation

Here are simple steps to prepare us to meditate.

1. Set Aside 30 Minutes per Day

To help get in the habit and increase our skill levels quickly, we set aside 30 minutes per day, at least 5 days per week for a minimum of 4 weeks. After that, we can reduce the frequency if we wish. We may not meditate the whole 30 minutes initially; it may only be for 10 minutes. But if I said let's meditate for 10 minutes, we'd keep looking at our watch – or phone – waiting for the time to be up, which makes the mind hard to settle in the now. Is the time up yet? No. Is the time up yet? No. I think you get the idea. By giving ourselves plenty of time, we offer our mind permission and make it easier to be here and now.

2. Choose a Quiet Place

We need a place to meditate to sit, knowing we won't be disturbed for the half hour. It doesn't have to be perfectly quiet; I meditate regularly in a house on a noisy street. We meditate more easily if we know no one will disturb us.

3. Remove Distractions

Turn off mobile phones, tablets, TVs, music – anything that might be a distraction. If we are expecting a call or a knock on the door at any time, then our mind will not let us focus on the now; it will be in the future waiting for the call or knock at any moment. If our family needs reminding, we can put up a do not disturb sign and teach them what it means; it's only for half an hour.

4. Use a Comfortable Seat

We don't lay down. Why? We will fall asleep rather than meditate. Ideally, we sit on a chair or a set of cushions. An office chair will do. We need to feel comfortable enough to sit in the chair for 30 minutes without moving but not so comfortable that we doze off.

5. Have Nothing Moving

Nothing should be in our vision that can distract us, especially anything moving, such as incense smoke, candles or mobiles – mini sculptures – dangling from the ceiling. If we want them in the room, we try to keep them out of sight.

6. Commit

We must make sure that no matter how we feel when we wake up or how we feel during the day, we do the meditation if that is what we have committed to. If we give our mind even the slightest chance of getting out of the meditation – do what it feels like rather than what we commit to – then the moment things aren't going so well, we will stop. By committing – no matter what – we activate acceptance and slip into our routine more quickly. We must do what we say. If we say that we will do it, then we make sure we do. Otherwise, we don't commit to it in the first place.

7. Sit and Breathe

At the beginning of each session, we sit down comfortably and take a few long and slow breaths. Make the time to let ourselves settle down.

* * * * *

Our preparation is now complete. Wasn't so bad, was it? Don't worry if it doesn't come naturally. It will, with practice.

The Skill

Here are four types of meditations or practices of mindfulness. I recommend you read through all of them then choose one to practise – the one you feel might work best. Then practise it and practise it. If one doesn't work well, try another. There isn't one that everyone prefers. If you wish, learn a few and be good at each; it will give you more tools in your tool chest to use when you need them most, such as having to calm down quickly – as can happen in an important meeting or just before an interview, performance or exam. Don't give up on any of them too quickly. It can take time to get used to them and for them to work well for us, but once we have mastered them enough, we can find them invaluable.

Don't worry; the meditations aren't complicated. In fact, we'll start with the simplest one first.

Mindfulness Skill 1. Zen-type Meditation

I have been doing this meditation for years. I taught myself almost accidentally. Then I read many years later it is like what Zen meditation specialists or masters do – hence the name.

Like all the following meditations, it assumes we have followed the preparations described above. Please make sure you have completed them; they really help.

Steps for Zen-type Meditation

Sit and Stare

Sit in your chair or on your cushions. Find a place in front of you to stare at comfortably. It can be a mark on a door or a spot on the wall or floor or in a corner. Please don't look at paintings, complex pictures or designs, as your eyes will be tempted to wander; we don't want that.

Keep Still

The aim is to keep perfectly still and keep staring. We are allowed to do two things. First, we can breathe – or we will pass out. Second, we can blink – or we will get eye ulcers. Other than breathing and blinking, we keep still for as long as possible – at least 10 to 15 minutes.

No Eye Movement

This is important: we should not move our eyes, not even a little. Why? When we start thinking about a problem, what do our eyes do? They move. Keeping our eyes still allows our minds to focus on what we are looking at. At the same time, not moving our eyes settles our thoughts. It's too hard to think and keep our eyes still at the same time.

Be in the Zone

The brain is used to noticing our movements (such as head turning) and the many changes in what we see (such as people walking past). Once we stop most of the input and keep it the same, the brain tends to settle. Some know this as getting into the zone. It may take 10 or 15 minutes at first. If we keep still and focused, our mind will eventually and naturally chill, which is what we want.

Many people tell me they like this meditation because it is so simple. Those busy bees who must keep physically moving and hate sitting still – like Kallie always on the go – notice it a challenge. I find it a great way of settling the mind before contemplative meditation and exploring the subtleties of deeper emotions.

I believe Zen masters can keep this mediation going for hours, days or longer. I think that is a waste of time, but each to their own. For us to gain benefits, 20 to 30 minutes is just fine.

Mindfulness Skill 2. Fish in a Stream

This is a meditation I learned from a colleague who teaches it to her clients. It focuses more on giving us skills to help manage our thoughts. As with all our meditations, it assumes we have completed the preparations we mentioned earlier.

Steps for Fish in a Stream

Sit with Eyes Open or Closed

Sit as we have before with eyes either open or closed – your choice. Many find it easier with their eyes closed. Don't worry if your eyes wander a little.

Imagine Your Thoughts as Fish in a Stream

Imagine you are on the bank of a stream. In the creek are fish swimming past you. Imagine these are your thoughts. You are just observing them.

Don't Engage

Let the thoughts pass by; just observe them, don't analyse them or focus on them in any way. Our mind usually reels in the thought, and we give it lots of attention and get emotionally engaged with it. Here we don't want any engagement at all; just observe them.

Throw the Fish Back

If you find a thought that has your attention imagine taking it off the hook and throwing it back in with all the other thoughts to let it swim on by. No matter how critical the thought might be, let it go. If it is important enough, it will show up once we have finished, and we will deal with it then. Just sit and observe.

Keep Detached

If fish in a stream isn't your thing, then you might like to imagine your thoughts as small wooden boats floating by. Some visualise their thoughts on the other side of frosted glass, which isn't clear to see through. If one thought becomes more apparent and we engage with it, we throw it back over the glass to pass by with the others. The key is to observe, not get emotionally involved in the thought, notice it detached from you, and stay there.

I taught this once to a lady who worked in a post office, and this was her favourite. First, she imagined thoughts in parcel boxes. Then, when a thought had her attention, she imagined putting the thought in a box, putting it on a conveyor belt beside her, and off it went to join the others. Brilliant.

This is a great skill to allow us to take a step back from our feelings, especially fears. Letting us be the observer will enable us to stop the fear from taking control and help us to be less reactive. In addition, it will allow us to tame our fears wherever we are.

Mindfulness Skill 3. The Off Switch

This meditation/mindfulness skill is the equivalent of finding the mind's off switch; here it is! I taught myself this one as a uni student.

It was in the early years of study, and I was pushing my mind as much as possible. After a while, my mind started to fog, and learning became harder the more I tried. So, one day I found a quiet place, closed my eyes, and discovered a way to switch it off. After a few minutes, my mind felt refreshed entirely, and I could learn more efficiently and think more clearly.

Steps for the Off Switch

Sit with Eyes Closed
Sit comfortably. Close your eyes. Take a few slow breaths.

Imagine a Deep Well
Imagine inside you is a deep well. At the bottom of the well is the real you: a person who is wise and all-knowing. There is gradual darkness between you and the bottom that gets darker the further you look down. The darkness – a nothingness; nothing is there, not even emotions – is perfectly calm and safe, calmer and safer the further you look down.

Float and Immerse
Imagine floating down into the nothingness and being completely immersed in it. The deeper you go, the more your thoughts and feelings drift away and are absorbed by the dark. Finally, you become the soft and peaceful nothingness. All thoughts and feelings are replaced by the void. Your whole being becomes nothing. If you notice a thought or feeling, it means you have floated back up. Gently float down again, deeper and deeper, immersing yourself in nothing where no thought or feeling exists.

Rest Without a Care or Thought

Guide yourself ever deeper into your safe and quiet nothingness. If you struggle to visualise the void, think of it as a peaceful and empty blackness; there is nothing in it. That is how I imagine it: as a darker and darker blackness where nothing exists.

The further down you float, the less you notice of anything – nothing exists in this darkness/nothingness, no care or thought. If you feel the sensation of your body floating as you practise this, do not be alarmed; it is perfectly normal.

*****

As we've noted – and Stan was noticing – the mind is always busy and never rests. Even at night, we are busy dreaming, whether or not we remember the dreams. So, by focusing on blackness/nothingness and immersing ourselves in it, we force our minds to consciously stop. This gives us no reaction or problem to see, no cause to consider what is bothering us; we offer our minds a rest.

Some people don't like the idea of using darkness or blackness in this meditation. They relate darkness to evil and light to good. That is up to them. Personally, I find the light is noisy and dark is empty and quiet, a place to get away from everything and rest. For me, darkness or blackness is neither good nor bad; it just is. Perhaps if you find darkness too unsettling you might change the blackness for a deeply soothing colour, such as blue or green. Float down and totally immerse yourself in this colour as described above.

With practice, once you have mastered this meditation, you will find you can bring your mind into that calming place and what it feels like in seconds, no matter where you are. It is a powerful fear-taming technique.

Mindfulness Skill 4. Focus on the Breath

There are many ways to use breathing to calm ourselves – to tame our fear. You may have already learned a few; breathing techniques are very popular for relaxing us. Using breathing to bring our minds to the present is easy to do. We will recommend breathing techniques specific to helping end a panic attack in a moment.

Steps for Focus on the Breath

Sit Comfortably

We sit as recommended in the preparation. Eyes can be open or closed. We will not be focusing on our thoughts.

Breathe

Take a few regular, slow breaths: not so slow that we gasp for air, and not so fast we get lightheaded, but something comfortable and in between.

Focus Attention

As you breathe, notice the air moving in and out. Notice it coming in through your nostrils, down the back of the throat, and down your windpipe behind your breastbone. Notice your chest expanding and your abdomen moving out as you breathe in. In and out. In and out. Notice the chest fall and the abdomen retreat as you breathe out.

Focus Feeling

Now focus your attention on one area where you notice the breath. It can be the nostrils, the throat, the chest – anywhere you can feel the breath. First, notice what the breath feels like at just that one place in your body. Then, notice more and more of what you can feel in that one body location with each breath in and out.

You Are the Breath

There is nothing but the breath and where you feel it. All your focus is on the breath. Feel and notice that feeling of each breath more with every slow breath in and out, in and out. Notice the feeling, recognise something new each time in that one location in your body, every breath in and every breath out. Try to feel and notice as much as you can with each breath.

The more we focus entirely on the breath, the more the mind is present in the now and calm; it can't focus on other things. Fear is tamed.

This was a favourite meditation of a businessman who came to see me. He found he would get very nervous before big meetings that involved dealings in the millions; the fear would cloud his thoughts. By focusing on his breath, initially outside before the meeting and later while in it if needed, his mind cleared. He could settle well and keep mentally sharp without being overwhelmed with fear.

* * * *

PANIC ATTACKS

This is an excellent opportunity to talk about how to control panic attacks since panic attacks can often be settled with breathing changes.

Panic attacks are an extreme form of the fear reaction. Typical panic attack symptoms include a racing heart, agitation and sweaty palms. These are like common fear symptoms. But what often scares people the most about panic is the lightheadedness to the point of feeling they will pass out. There are also pins and needles in the tips of the fingers and toes and around the lips. Many feel they are having a stroke or heart attack and are convinced they will die. We don't die from panic, by the way.

During panic, we tend to over-breathe. You may know this as sighing regularly or feeling you can't get enough breath. Some people mistake panic for an asthma attack. Chest tightness and shortness of breath can be extreme.

Most of the distressing symptoms of panic are because we over-breathe, which lowers our blood carbon dioxide. This changes our blood pH – its acidity. The brain reads the change in pH as indicating we aren't getting enough oxygen. So, we breathe more. Soon we are in a cycle of over-breathing and feeling worse and worse.

The key then is to allow our carbon dioxide levels to rise. In the past, many would recommend putting a paper bag around the lips and then breathe in and out into the bag. A more straightforward way is to alter our breathing.

> For instance, we count to seven as we slowly breathe in. We hold our breath for the same count of seven. Then breathe out over a count of fourteen at the same smooth rate. We do this three times in a row without any deep breaths in between. The numbers to remember are 7-7-14. If you count slowly, it could be 5-5-10. Holding our breath and breathing out slowly during this exercise allows carbon dioxide to build up. Breathing out gradually also slows our heart rate and calms us further.
>
> Many breathing techniques can help settle panic. Talk to a therapist if you wish to learn more.

Choose which meditation you prefer and practise it. Don't expect instant results. I have heard it said that meditation is best considered as a muscle. If you don't use it, it gets all flabby and unhealthy and wastes away. Keep using it, and we have the strength to call on whenever we need it.

* * * * *

Do I still practise any of these meditations?

I still use them at various times. However, I now prefer a deeper form of meditation that allows access to the symphony of feelings well beyond the obvious ones, such as fear, anger, hate, annoyance and frustration. Consider, if you wish, these simple meditations as an introduction to developing an ability to connect with your deeper self and all its subtleties. That is what I use meditation for. Meditation is a great skill to help tame our fear and settle us when we need it.

Other mindfulness suggestions

Are there other ways to bring the mind into the present without meditation? Yes. Consider the following, some of which you may also wish to try.

Speak What You Notice

Spend a moment when no one is around saying everything you notice, everything you see, smell, hear and feel. Notice as much of the present as you can. For example, I can see the picture on the wall, smell the air freshener, feel the weight of my hand resting on my leg. I can hear a person walking across the street and smell the lavender flowers near the fence I walk by. Notice as much as you can, in as much detail as you can. Do this for several minutes.

Adult Colouring In

Adult colouring in or painting can offer us enormous relief from our concerns by focusing our attention. There are many adult colouring-in-books and paint-by-numbers pictures available.

Mindfulness Apps

If you are into apps, then download one that helps promote mindfulness. Some clients have found them very helpful and use them regularly. I don't promote any type over another. See what works best for you.

Mindful Walk

Go for a 20-minute walk alone every day. During the walk, try to notice as many details as you can around you: the flowers, the grass, the fences, the houses, the road or path, and what is beside it. Focus on what you can and take it in; just notice and feel it. Don't take the dog or a partner; they will be too much of a distraction.

Make Mind-chill Your Thing

There are almost endless activities we can do to practise being mindful. First, we need to remember that our aim is to bring our minds firmly into the present. By doing so, we tame fear and significantly reduce our fear burden. Then life develops a calmer feel to it. Along the way, we might notice more of life and feel more immersed in it.

* * * * *

Stan preferred to try the Off Switch meditation. He also started regular walking or running – well known to settle our minds and reduce our anxiety. Soon, his thoughts weren't so hard to control anymore. He felt confident he wasn't going crazy. Within weeks he was already feeling so much better.

Thankfully, Covid restrictions around the world have eased. The world is opening up. If a new variant arises and we have little immunity, this may change with short notice. Being at home more may be the new way of life for some of us. This is an excellent opportunity to better manage and guide our minds, to feel settled with our thoughts. However, if when alone we feel restless, agitated and on edge and our mind won't stop, what better time to go for a mindful walk, practise a mindfulness activity or sit down and find relief in mindfulness meditation. Whether or not Covid is impacting our lives, these mindfulness techniques offer potent ways to reduce our overall fear burden.

* * * * *

Next we will learn practical strategies to help reduce our fears related to being too busy.

CHAPTER 5

TAME THE BUSY

Stage 3. Shift From Busy to Happy, Manageable and Chilled

Are you one of those people who needs to be on the go all the time, never a moment's rest? Does this unrelenting busyness exhaust you? Does it increase your stress to breaking point? Does it all seem too much and too overwhelming? Perhaps Covid has made you busier still, with home schooling and higher demands put on you by family, friends or work. Being too busy can be an enormous fear burden to carry, as Belinda came to realise.

Belinda was an amazingly fast, efficient and capable nurse I worked with in Sydney many years ago. She was sometimes playfully called a busy bee, always on the go. It was great for the practice: stuff got done. We didn't realise her busyness was a symptom of unmanaged anxiety. One day Belinda shared with us her psychologist's recommendation: to make time to sit down for a proper breakfast each morning rather than just grab what she could on the way to work. Belinda shared that making that time to quietly sit and eat breakfast at the table made all the difference to her anxiety; it started her day without rushing. It was a decisive first step to reducing her personal torment with stress.

As Belinda had begun to find out, slowing down was a powerful and simple way to tame fear.

In our effort to reduce our fear burden, slowing down has two main benefits:

- It tames fears directly.
- It gives the brain the moments it needs to tame its fear.

There is a quality of our fear response we didn't focus on earlier: fear helps us speed up. It is one reason why a racing car driver's heart is the fastest you will see in any sport. Their fear response keeps them sharp and quick when they are behind the wheel. Slow down our busy lives and, like Belinda, we automatically reduce – tame – any fear keeping us in the fast lane.

The other way slowing down helps us to tame fear is giving us time.

We now know our brain needs a plan or acceptance to resolve fears, but coming up with these takes conscious moments to think about them. How can our brain be expected to deal with all its worries if it never gets those moments? Yes, setting aside worry time – see above – can help, but so too does slowing down our life so we have periods to think and just ponder. How many fast and busy people do you know who have time to ponder? Kallie, we noted earlier, indeed wasn't getting any pondering moments for reflection.

Like it or not, living life constantly on the go, as Belinda and Kallie were, is not suitable for helping to tame and control our fears and anxieties.

Does that mean slowing down will be easy?

Not if busy is our habit or drive. For Belinda, it became a habit; she slipped into it without realising it. Pulling back from being hectic didn't seem easy. For someone like Kallie, not going full speed would be as foreign as living alone on the moon: not easy at all.

Should we choose to slow down, it can be expected to not feel natural at first. But with practice, we can find enormous ongoing relief and a significant reduction in our fear burden.

How to Slow Down and Still Feel OK

How can we tame fear by slowing down without increasing our worry that something hasn't been done, without fear of missing out (FOMO)?

Consider the following measures. If you aren't a busy person, you will still find these skills helpful.

Measure 1. An Activity Diary

Our first task is to see how busy we are and where we spend our time. Often we underestimate what we do if we rely on memory alone. Try this instead.

Keep an activity diary for a week.

- For one week, keep a journal of everything you do and how much time it takes. I don't like logs either, but this is only for seven days. It will be worth it.
- List the time for sleep, breakfast, getting ready for work, travel, work, the other activities of your day, then the evening activities. List them all. You may find it helpful to use a diary or small pocket notebook – like your worry book – or an app.
- Write the list in shorthand or abbreviations, so it doesn't take too much time; for example, 'Bfst 10mins' to note breakfast

time, 'Slp 6hrs' to signify sleep time, '2work 40mins' to denote travel to work, and so on.
- Make a habit of writing in your diary what you have done each time you finish an activity or soon after. Don't leave it to the vagaries of imperfect memory.

Now, at the end of the day, use a big red marker or pen to circle the times when you were particularly nervous, worried or afraid.

How do your week and days look? Busy? Nervous?

Now we work on how to change it.

Measure 2. An Essentials List

Before we consider changing anything, we need to know what is essential. List the seven most important things you value in your life – your most important priorities.

My priorities

1. ....
2. ....
3. ....
4. ....
5. ....
6. ....
7. ....

If you can't find seven, that's OK; write down what you can. Don't share this list with your partner or anyone else, not yet. This is for you and you alone to create. For instance, a typical list might include the kids, spouse, finances, success, health, job satisfaction, friends, extended family and regular holidays. It isn't for me to pre-empt you; write down what you feel from your heart is honestly driving you in your life. There are no right or wrong answers.

Measure 3. Do They Mesh?

Compare your two lists: your activity list and your priority list.

- How well do the two lists match?
- If your kids are high on your priority list, how much time did you spend with them in activities?
- If your spouse or partner is a top priority, when was the last time you spent one-on-one time with them chatting or having fun?
- How much sleep did you get if your health is a major priority?
- If family and friends are most important, did you spend enough time with them compared to work?
- If success at work is essential, how much quality time did you spend making your ambitions happen?

In short, did your priorities list line up with the times you spent in the activities of your week?

It is common for our claimed values and priorities to not match our actions, just like Kallie and her regret. She said the family and children were her priority, and yet her actions said work clearly came first. It took Covid to remind her that her priorities and actions didn't align.

Why did we do this exercise?

There were two main reasons:

- to help us align our life with our values to feel better about ourselves and where we are heading
- most importantly, to help us see where we can cut back so we don't get so upset when we no longer do all that stuff we really don't need to do.

Before we get too nervous, our aim isn't to stop doing everything except eat and sleep and indulge in a few other joys. No, instead of doing a hundred things we don't have time for, the purpose is to cut it back to eighty that we can do comfortably and still have time to reflect so our brain can chill.

How do we cut back and know what to give up doing?

Measure 4. Take Time to Make Time

If we are going to cut back on activities, we need to know what we can give up. A simple way to help us identify this is to understand the minimums we need to live a satisfying life. Then, if we want to add activities to that and we have the time to do so, that's great.

How do we know what these minimums are?

I have found that the table titled A Balance for Parents from my book *A Balance of Self* (Vivid, Fremantle, 2011) offers a great list of minimum needs for all of us to consider when trying to 'tame the busy'. It can be a helpful guide even if we don't have children at home. If, for example, you are single and need to balance work, study and volunteering. In that case, you vary your hours according to your priorities. Consider the following.

A BALANCE FOR PARENTS

TIME	ACTIVITY	AIM OR REASON	HUMAN ESSENCE
1-2hrs/wk	Quiet time	Be in the moment Listen to self	Personal self
1-2hrs/wk	Enjoyment time	Connect with self Have fun	Personal self
1 evening or night/wk	One-on-one couples time, e.g. dinner out No kids Time to talk	Relationship maintenance Build and maintain friendship	Family self
1 weekend every second month	One-on-one couples time	Relationship maintenance Fulfil relationship needs	Family self
2-3 x 1-hr sessions/wk	One-on-one parent and child time No disturbances by others for at least 1 hr	Have fun Play at child's level doing what they like	Family self Personal self
2-3 hrs/wk	Time with friends only	Male-male and female-female bonding Talk Have fun	Community self
1 lunch or dinner per month	Time with extended family to socialise	Build family ties and supports Share problems and good times	Family self
< 40 hrs/wk	Work/job	Income	Community self

What does this table teach us?

The table is based on the needs summarised by the Balance of Self Model (see the book *A Balance of Self* and Appendix 1). This model has four components. It breaks our needs into three basic human needs of self:

- our individual needs
- our family needs — the requirements to have, and be part of, a family
- the community needs — to have friends we can trust; we are social beings, after all.

In the centre of the model is land, essentially nature. The Balance for Parents table offers an example of how we might balance our time between these needs, offering minimum times to build our life around. For example, we must have self time of at least several hours per week. We must also make time to connect with our family and friends. Work, you will notice, is limited to less than 40 hours per week.

The recommendations can also be seen to contain many fear-taming strategies. For example, the table emphasises the need for each of us to have quiet time. We can use this time to chill and practise mindfulness (see above).

One-on-one time with our partner helps maintain a close friendship — lessening the fear of breaking up. A common reason we break up is we lose the intimate connection. It is hard to keep that connection if we barely talk.

One-on-one parent time with children helps increase their self-worth and certainty that we care. It helps them feel safe, reducing their stress and fear.

Friendships with same-sex mates and girlfriends also help us feel more secure, knowing there are others we can call on when we are in need. We will look more into using connection to tame social anxieties in Chapter 7.

Similarly, by spending time with extended family and ensuring we get along, our children can feel more secure – less afraid. They know they will always have an extended family to call on when needed.

And, finally, by working fewer than 40 hours, we give ourselves time to live a balanced life, relax, slow down and spend more quality time with those we love and cherish most.

As we have seen, finding the balance in life that works best for us also just happens to become a fear-reducing exercise.

What about extracurricular activities for the kids, such as sports or music lessons?

In the scheme of things, it would be hard to disagree that what children need most is socialising with friends and playing (preferably outside) – children learn much from play. And they all need to develop friendship skills so they don't become lonely, angry, depressed adults. But, beyond that, if the extra activities stop any of us from meeting the basics, then maybe they need to go. We don't want to be so caught up in additional activities with the kids that it stresses us all out or doesn't let us slow down, do we?

But I don't have enough family and supports to get one-on-one time. What do I do?

Then perhaps we need a trusted professional babysitter once a week? Finally, if we have recently moved into a new suburb and there is no family support or if we don't have the capacity to pay a babysitter maybe it's time to network to support each other.

I remember someone telling me that the three most important things for a relationship when the kids come along are babysitter, babysitter and babysitter. He and his wife would call a babysitter once a week so they could go out and just talk. It is a brilliant strategy. It helped keep them close. Of course, great if you can afford it.

Let's be honest, most of the time we are extra busy because of choice rather than circumstance. If we must work two full-time jobs to pay for the rent and food, that is a rotten break; it shouldn't be like that. Having said that, many of us stress ourselves needlessly by overcommitting, often financially. We don't need the huge mortgage that drives us to work insane hours to pay it off, but we choose it. It's for the children's future, we say. It's to get ahead. I need this!

Do we?

I get it; it's hard to cut back on a lifestyle once we are used to it. But where was lifestyle on our priority list? Was it above our health or the health and wellbeing of our family? Was it above our children's emotional wellbeing and sense of security; their need for us to love and guide them?

Ask yourself the question honestly, can we cut back? Discuss it with your partner and family if they are involved. Would cutting back relieve some of the pressure? Do we need more assistance to get by? Do we need help? Don't feel embarrassed.

Sadly, the way of western life is to be increasingly self-sufficient and do it alone. This can leave us disconnected and feeling ashamed to ask for help. Yet, working together, we can cut back costs and stress. For example, instead of sending children to childcare, why not get to know the other mums in the area and see if you can share the babysitting, create a creche group?

Of course, suppose we had more significant government and/or community support. In that case, we could spend more time with our children and friends while still having a meaningful job – just saying. Maybe we should talk to our local members about raising social support for those struggling to meet the basics. It would be a powerful way to reduce our fear burden. Perhaps for the same reason we should be prioritising creating a more supportive community.

Other suggested ways to slow down:

- Make time to eat a meal, as Belinda learned. Never eat – let alone do make-up – on the run.
- Don't watch TV or do other activities during main meals. Ideally, sit down to your meal with others and talk.
- Take more time when eating your meals. Eat more slowly.
- Cook more slow food. Take time to prepare food instead of buying fast food.
- Instead of rushing through each day at 100 miles an hour, cut it back to 70 miles an hour and notice how that feels. Try it for one day as a trial. Then, imagine going just a bit slower every day, and do it.
- When you find yourself rushing, stop and spend a minute taking a few slow and calming breaths.
- Make quality sleep your absolute priority. Get at least seven to eight hours – no excuses. If you find you can't sleep, seek professional help, such as consulting your family doctor.

Slowing down can be challenging – I get it – but it can also be gratifying and calming. So perhaps, like Belinda, we need to slow down one step at a time, like just making time for breakfast.

What if I find I just can't slow down? Even the thought makes me feel uncomfortable.

Then I recommend seeing a therapist. Like Kallie earlier, what may stop you is something you are hiding or running from that you haven't dealt with or recognised yet. It will be next to impossible for Kallie to tame her busy life while she continues to be scared not to be the success her father wanted her to be. Of course, she has every right to be driven by whatever motivations she chooses.

*****

Perhaps in the age of Covid, slowing down isn't as relevant to you as creating a less chaotic life. Chaos breeds uncertainty. Uncertainty, the unfamiliar, as we have seen, promotes fear.

In the following chapter we will learn to find calm and peace by building certainty.

CHAPTER 6

THE CALM FOUND IN CERTAINTY

Stage 4. Find Peace in the Predictable

'Are you saying Tim's going to be anxious like me? It's my fault?' Carol, a mother of five, asked emphatically. Tim was the second youngest and about to start high school. Carol had come to renew a medication for her anxiety and depression originally prescribed five years earlier. Soon we began to discuss the benefits of seeing a psychologist, such as to learn new skills so eventually she could get off the drugs; she didn't want to be on them forever. She would occasionally touch her short brown hair that seemed randomly styled, a natural look. We began to talk about how anxiety often runs in families. I inadvertently mentioned how her learning new skills to manage her anxiety would benefit her children, including Tim. She looked like I'd thrown dirt in her face. Not a smart move on my part.

In my defence, and in hindsight, my mistake was that I didn't get to know Carol well before I discussed a topic that clearly triggered needs in her to be a faultless mum. The truth was she had – unwittingly – contributed to Tim's anxiety, as anxious parents are likely to do whether they are aware of it or not. So how was she contributing to the anxiety? What didn't she want to hear?

When I mentioned that life must be busy with such a big family, Carol was happy to share how busy. As Carol had described it, family life was on the go all the time: instrument lessons here, soccer practice there. The youngest wants to stay over at a friend's place, a new drama between disagreeing children erupts at any time. And between all this, she was working part time; what else can we do? We get by. Getting by, I also learned, meant the family had meals when they could; there was no sit-down breakfast, lunch or dinner. In addition, the children were expected to brush their teeth, have a shower and get to bed at whatever hour they wanted, so long as it wasn't too late. Weekends were random; between all the sports the children were chauffeured to by parents, everyone did what they felt like, except on family birthdays when everyone had to attend. To me, Carol was describing chaos. What surprised me was that only Tim was suffering anxiety like his mother. If I'd been in that house, I'd have been a nervous wreck. Thankfully, her husband never seemed to get flustered.

Yes, Carol and Tim's life was too busy. Still, on top of that, it lacked predictability, which was almost certainly a significant contributor to their anxiety – daily high levels of fear.

As we recently noted, an unpredictable world is a world filled with the unknown, the unfamiliar. And our brain reacts to the unfamiliar with a fear response – often known or felt as anxiety. So, the higher the uncertainty in our life, the higher the burden of fear we can expect to dominate it, like it was now doing for Carol and Tim.

Thankfully, predictability removes the unknown element; it is a potent way to tame fear.

How can we add predictability to our lives?

Two simple ways are through routine and structure. Children, especially, thrive on routine and structure. Tim, for instance, found he was less anxious at school, where he had rigorous timetables and routines.

But what about freedom to do what I like when I like it? I hate having to answer to others and do what they want all the time.

Here is the great battle we all must face. On the one hand, we crave choices and unlimited freedom – to do what we want when we want to. Yet, on the other hand, the more options and freedoms we give ourselves, the more uncertainty we bring and the more fear and anxiety; who knows what will happen next? Imagine a competitive world where it is everyone for themselves. Who knows when someone will attack us and take our stuff, including our food, maybe our life? In such a scenario the notion of everyone having total freedom is terrifying. So, we have less choice and limited freedoms – just the right balance – and we live far less stressful and anxious lives and feel safer.

Ideally, our structure and routine should be a choice. However, giving children unlimited choices doesn't work; their brain hasn't learned to see far enough into the future to understand the consequences of their actions. Therefore, it is up to parents to set the structure and boundaries and, within these, parents offer as many choices as is reasonable so that their children feel calm and secure.

A simple example of how to offer a choice for a child within a structure is to lay out three sets of clothes for them, and then they choose which one they would like to wear – no other choices. This gives them the feeling they aren't just being dictated to, and they can make choices too.

But by trying to make life predictable, haven't I just killed the wonderful spice of spontaneity? What about the unexpected, like the random candlelit dinner made for our partner when they come home, the spontaneous night away, or the last-minute choice of where we eat out or place to visit on the weekend?

Not at all. We can still enjoy spontaneity within the framework of a solid and reassuring structure and routine. Within the structure, spontaneity can still be well-nourished – my turn to choose where we go this weekend, remember, we agreed?

How can we create more structure and routine in our lives to tame our fear while preserving choice and spontaneity?

Consider the following methods.

Methods to Create Structure and Routine

Method 1. The Whiteboard

Buy a whiteboard to plan out your week. Organise the board as follows. This example is for a family, but it can be adapted to work just as well for someone living alone or for a couple without children at home.

- Draw in vertical columns for each day of the week, and horizontal columns representing the times (7am, 8am, etc.).
- Cross out set times (such as breakfast, lunch and dinner), so all family members know when they are and make time for them.
- Get everyone in the family to put in their self-times – times to do their own thing – and activities, such as sports and meeting friends.
- Put in your couple's time; when was the last time you went on a date?
- Put in your quiet time so everyone knows when not to disturb you.

- Put in one-on-one times with the children to play with them doing what they like – no screen time. The attention must be one on one; no one else can be there.
- Put in your mates'/girlfriends' time – time to be with friends.
- Put in family or recreation time to get away as a family or invite other extended family members over.
- Put in work.
- Put in other things you would like to do or get done.
- Leave spaces to fill in as you want on the day – your spontaneous times.

Done!

We have just created structure and routine. The trick, of course, is to follow it.

A mum once told me this works exceptionally well in her home. Her son suffers from mild to moderate autism. He gets distraught and anxious when he doesn't know what will happen. The whiteboard, prominent in the kitchen, means at any time he can see what everyone will be doing, and he becomes much calmer.

To help the structure work better, we can apply a few other tips:

- Don't plan things too tight; allow time to run late.
- Have plans in place if this ideal doesn't work – a plan B in case the plan A on the board doesn't work out; be flexible.
- Don't make changes to the plan without a complete family consultation unless it is an emergency.
- Ideally, set up the week's plan on just one day a week; for example, everyone does it together on a Sunday.

- Create times when a family member chooses what the rest does, like where to go on a family outing. This adds to everyone's sense of agency and increases their self-worth; they feel they contribute significantly.

There are many great benefits of this whiteboard other than just creating predictability:

- It shows children how to create a balanced life. It role-models how to be a functional parent. It lets children see what a balanced life looks like so they can use it as an example when they are an adult.
- It shows us what we are doing with our lives to see if we live according to our values and priorities. Am I really putting family first like I believe I should be?
- It helps us see that we are doing what we choose to. The list is our choice; no one has put a gun to our head to make us do it.
- It helps the family see everyone's times and activities are worthy of respect. We make times for everyone; everyone is important. It makes us more equal and dissuades favouritism.
- It brings families together in decision making. It can make us closer by working as a team and learning to compromise.
- It teaches our children how to ask and negotiate for what they want rather than have a tantrum or give up and be too submissive.
- It reduces behavioural problems in our children. So long as they get their say and have their one-on-one parent time, for instance, they don't need to misbehave for attention.

The idea of using a weekly whiteboard to create structure doesn't only work for families; it works for individuals. As an individual, the whiteboard structure can offer us a stable part of our life to build around, to calm the chaos. It can also provide us with meaning and purpose.

For example, I suggested to an anxious businessman starting his own business to use a weekly whiteboard with planned-out days and week. He found it invaluable. It stopped him from getting too distracted. It showed him what he was doing in his day and that he wasn't wasting time; he was productive. In addition, with just a glance at the whiteboard on the wall he could see where he needed to focus his attention next. He found this much better than an app on his phone or computer.

Of course, the whiteboard structure also works well with the worry book. So does a daily diary. For example, we can put in our following day activities from the worry book and lock them into our daily and weekly plan at the end of our day. Then, in our daily schedule, we can mark our breaks to pace ourselves; we all need rest.

A whiteboard is an invaluable tool for helping to create structure.

Method 2. Functional Habits

In my undergraduate years as a doctor-in-training, I remember one of our clinical teachers reminding us to treat every patient as an individual. He was against us simply treating them as an illness, a list of typical symptoms for a medical condition, such as shortness of breath and ankle swelling suggestive of heart failure. The patient is not Mr or Mrs heart failure. I get where he was coming from; he didn't want us to treat people as medical problems but as people. A decent idea; our patients are individuals and worthy of being treated as people. However, treating every case as unique made it hard to develop a quick and effective routine. When we're under the pump and behind in seeing patients, our functional habits and routines can save us. Following a list in our mind helps us be safe and effective. The last thing we want is a doctor to make a critical mistake; lives are on the line. So functional habits are our saving grace.

Functional habits are an excellent tool for reducing our burden of stress. I say 'functional' habits and not just any habits. If we have habits that harm us (such as drinking too much, smoking, or having regular unprotected sex) we add to the stress of getting sick. Oh, no, is the burning when I pee a sexually transmitted disease? Will it make me infertile?

Functional habits free us. They stop us from going over what we just did, repeatedly wondering if we did it right. For example, did I turn off the iron before I left? Did I lock the back door? Did I close the windows? Knowing we turn the iron off every time we are finished with it and we routinely lock the back door and close the windows when we leave frees us from worrying whether we did or not.

It was similar for me being a doctor-in-training. Having a routine of questions to consider and things to examine, test and follow up meant I could be sure – or as sure as I could be – I hadn't missed anything. It was a great relief and made being a doctor-in-training much less stressful. Those habits still do.

By having good habits, we can reassure ourselves we will do what works and reduce the thought in our mind that we will fail or have done it wrong. Whether at work or at home, functional habits reduce our fear burden at every turn.

How do we create functional habits?

Try the following:

- Create a list of activities you know are good for you, such as walking, eating proper meals, going to the gym, and shopping for ingredients rather than buying take out.
- Make regular times to fit in the suitable activities. For instance, I do workouts three times per week, walk three times a week and run at least once a week. In addition, I do my laundry in the evening of my last workday, so I have the rest of the weekend free.
- Create daily routines at work and at home, getting up at the same time each morning. Check your worry book at set times in the day. Clean up after cooking and dinner, rather than leaving it overnight. Make the bed as soon as you are up, and brush your teeth at least twice a day – if you aren't already. Once it's a routine, you don't have to think or worry about it.

If it's a complex task, such as filling out forms at work, then create a way to make it a routine so you can do the same thing repeatedly, knowing you will get it right.

How many activities could you make into a routine – a functional habit? Set aside half a day to think about it. Look at personal activities at home as well as work. You may be surprised how much less stress and anxiety you feel in your day by creating a functional routine.

We can all do with more functional habits.

Method 3. Know Your Job and Stick To It

It's hard to feel satisfied and confident in our job if we don't know what our job is.

I have seen many people suffer massive anxiety because they took on too much work that wasn't supposed to be their job anyway. This happened because their job wasn't well defined; there wasn't a clear job description. The other main reason was poor management – bosses not ensuring everyone was clear in their tasks and well supported.

A poor manager or management can make our life an uncertain, nervous hell. Aside from the fact they may have temper tantrums and take them out on us, they can make our job too big, unmanageable and unrealistic. On top of that, if they aren't supervising properly, they can let the better employees take up the slack of the lesser or struggling ones. One person's job soon becomes the job of one and a half, then two people's and maybe three. If we are scared to lose our job or don't like saying no, we can soon find our job terrifying. Next thing we start having nightmares about work and dread the thought of going to work the next day. I have had several clients this has happened to in different organisations, both private and in the government.

Whether at work or home, it is essential you know your job, what is expected of you and each other, and not take on too much – yes, mums too. To help you create this level of job or task certainty, try the following.

At Work

- Make sure you have a written copy of your job description and regularly check with management that it hasn't changed.
- If you are being asked to do more than you can reasonably cope with, be prepared to say no.
- Don't be scared to lose your job. Have a resume ready and be prepared to upskill if you need to so you don't feel trapped in the job you are in; keep yourself employable.
- Create routines and functional habits so you know you're doing your job well.

- If you are unsure whether you're doing the job to the standard expected, ask the boss early; don't leave yourself feeling uncertain.
- Use your worry book regularly and make sure to use your worry time.
- If the boss is unreasonable or abusive, talk to higher management. If they don't help, or they ignore or dismiss you, look higher still. I have supported patients as whole departments were dismissed because management didn't do their jobs and care for their staff. If going to the top doesn't work, then perhaps you need to change who you work for.

No job should leave us an anxious, scared mess. We must do our utmost to ensure we feel comfortable and secure in the position being asked of us.

At Home

- Have an open discussion about sharing the jobs around the house.
- Know what your partner expects of you. Don't assume you know; ask.
- Being subjected to abuse – physical, emotional or otherwise – is never OK. Seek help from professional health services early if you need them.
- Don't be afraid to say no if it needs to be said.
- Work as a team. One person's problem is everyone's problem, so no one should be blamed and everyone should work to fix it.
- Share what stresses you early. Never let it simmer. It isn't weak to share a worry; it is a sign of strength. (However, adults

shouldn't share adult problems, such as relationship or financial issues, with their children.)
- Regularly offer praise and support. We all feel better knowing we are doing well.
- Allow others to have different views. Respect each other's differences. It is OK to agree to disagree.

By ensuring we know what is expected of us, we give our life certainty. Certainty reduces fear. We all benefit if we keep our jobs and expectations of each other reasonable and achievable.

Method 4. Tradition

One of our family traditions is always meeting up for each other's birthday and for major public holidays, such as Christmas and Easter, and special occasions like Mother's Day and Father's Day. I know families who take traditional holidays at special places, like a resort, local island or coastal caravan park. Other families have regular big traditional get-togethers. Sure, meet-ups may seem ordinary at times or heated, depending on how the family gets along. Still, inherent in them are fundamentals that reduce our fears.

Traditions are especially powerful for children. As we've seen, children need, but also thrive on, predictability. Tradition builds on the rock of certainty. It further grounds children and adults.

Traditions such as giving presents, making food together or just having a yarn with a few jokes and games mixed in become something we look forward to. They also create a long-term functional habit that can be passed on down generations with benefits for all.

What about teenagers? As they get older, children often frown on traditions and want to spend more time with their friends or on the computer.

It is true, in the teen years the desire to fit in with peers is strong, and so teenagers can resent being tied to functions where they won't be with friends. But they should be encouraged to participate. It is worth remembering – perhaps this has happened to you – that often we don't fully appreciate the values of tradition until we are much older, especially when we have children of our own.

How do we increase tradition in our life?

We embrace the traditions handed down according to our culture. We invite others to join us in our celebrations. We make traditions a greater priority in our life. And if we don't have many traditions, we start to make them now, especially if we have a young family.

Set aside a day and sit down as a family to ask everyone what traditions they would like to have for the family. Let everyone have an equal say – no one talking over another. All ideas are on the table, and there are no good or bad ideas. Do you all want to go camping once a year or perhaps have a big end-of-season feast to get everyone together? Encourage everyone to be part of powerful family traditions they would be proud to hand down to their children and beyond.

Traditions are often ancient. They have continually stood the test of time because of their benefits. Traditions remain a powerful way to reduce our fear burden across a lifetime and beyond.

* * * * *

Unfortunately, Carol decided not to see me again after the session where she took offence; she now sees a colleague at the practice. Over the years, however, I have enjoyed helping many other families reduce their fear burden by creating a predictable structure and routine. They do work. The difficulty, as with Carol, is sharing the benefits in a way that doesn't appoint any blame. Fix ourselves, and we often fix our children. Suffering fear and passing our anxieties onto the generations after us isn't anyone's fault. However, once we know how to tame our fears, doesn't it become our responsibility to tame them in us, so our children don't suffer them too?

* * * * *

Covid has wreaked havoc on our social lives. Many of us were already struggling to connect, make friends and build relationships. Then Covid came along and made it two hundred times worse. For many of us, the only social connection we had was with colleagues at work. That was taken away too. The less we connect, the more anxious we can become. Isolation feeds social anxiety for reasons that we will look at soon. Whether isolated or alone, we can reduce a significant fear burden through connection. We will discuss how we might do this next.

CHAPTER 7

CONNECTION REDEMPTION

Stage 5. Find Peace in Connection

Brian was kindly referred to me by a practice colleague to see if I could help him with anxiety. Numerous psychologists and a few psychiatrists had failed. Grey short hair, a short grey beard and a stomach Homer Simpson would be proud of, Brian didn't only seem anxious but down. He'd started to believe nothing could help him. He was in his late fifties and in a stable relationship with a very understanding and caring partner. They both had grown-up children from past relationships who didn't pose any significant stress. Finances weren't a problem either; he worked for a government agency that offered a generous salary and retirement package. The problem was he felt too anxious to go to work. There was no apparent reason; everyone was amicable. There was no mistreatment, yet the mere thought of walking through the office doors sent uncontrollable shivers up his spine and sickness in the pit of his stomach. We sat down over a few sessions, and Brian filled me in. Covid hadn't helped.

Brian shared he'd had some form of social anxiety – being afraid to be around other people – since early school. As a child he'd had to wear a leg brace for years, and the bullying he suffered was heartbreaking.

Brian eventually found enjoyment in computers and software development. IT became his career. He gained some confidence making a few friends as he gained his qualifications and early experience. This gave him enough self-assurance to apply for a sought-after government job and get it. He told me getting that job was one of the proudest moments of his life. Brian said that for a long time, he'd been doing fine. Then Covid hit. Government departments were shut down or had to run on minimum staff. Brian was told he could do his job from home, so he did. For almost eighteen months, he could avoid just about everyone except family. Then they asked everyone to start to come back in. He was terrified.

Like Brian, many of us are scared or even terrified at the mere thought of being around others; social anxiety is a widespread fear. It is easy to feel scared of making a fool of ourselves, afraid of not fitting in. Not unusually, we can be scared we are phony and will be discovered. The latter is also known as imposter syndrome. When fear of others gets terrible enough, it is often given names like social phobia or agoraphobia. Social anxieties can quickly get so bad that we struggle to use public transport, attend work or go shopping. We can be terrified to meet new people, be in crowds or even leave our homes. Social anxiety, at its worst, can turn our house into a prison. For Brian, by now he was afraid of being around just about anyone, except those he knew well. He said even coming to the surgery and sitting in the waiting room was torture. Work just happened to be the social place he now feared the most. It didn't make sense to him; he knew, at least on a rational level, he would be safe there.

Why do so many of us, like Brian, have social fears?

The answer, in short, is it's a natural response.

It doesn't seem natural. After all, aren't we supposed to be social beings connected with others?

Yes, we are, but nature is peculiar about those we should strive to be around. It made us find safety and security among close friends and colleagues; we were made to be tribal.

Tribes are built on the idea that we all need each other to survive. We stay together because we know we all have each other's back, no matter what. Together, we enjoy the warm comfort of feeling safe among friends.

In other words, if we meet people we don't know and can't predict – those not of our tribe – then nature has decided we should treat them like a possible threat; they aren't close, so they might harm or kill us. So, once again, the brain is using the cautious approach of better overreact and survive than underreact and die; at least we can be sure our close friends will be safe.

We develop social anxiety primarily because being afraid of others can quickly spiral out of control.

Imagine we start to get afraid of people around us. Perhaps we feel we don't fit in or that others aren't being as kind as we would like, as Brian experienced as a kid. What do we do then? We avoid these nasty people and others too. If one group of people is threatening, what's stopping everyone else from doing the same? But that act of avoidance creates a reaction: our social anxiety worsens, raising our general level of fear with it.

How does that work?

It is well known that when we are away from the safety of those we trust, our overall fear and arousal levels go up. It has been documented, for example, that people who feel alone have shorter reaction times to possible threats. When we are in a tribe, we have many eyes to watch out for danger, like looking out for prowling big hungry beasts. If one of us sees it, we all soon know about it. But if we are alone, there aren't as many eyes to watch our back. It means we must be more vigilant, more afraid. So now we aren't just nervous about others; we are edgy about everything. Even noises we'd otherwise not worry about can set us off.

Do you worry about every bump in the night or the car backfiring but without a good reason?

The good news is the more we hang around people, the more predictable they become. We get to know how they'll react to losing a job, breaking up, meeting other people and taking risks or if we sit in their seat or question their political views. How many friends or people do you know so well that for you they are predictable?

As we now know, the brain increases our fear when faced with the unfamiliar. The more we stay away from people, the more foreign they become and the more afraid we feel, even among those we once called our friends or work acquaintances, as was the case for Brian. He was never close to these people at work. Still, he started to feel they were predictable by regularly being around them. Once he left for an extended time, it was like everyone was unfamiliar again. It understandably made him afraid.

Put simply, social anxiety/fears are our brain's way of asking: where's my tribe?

* * * * *

Before we continue, it is crucial to realise our social anxiety and feeling lonely and that we don't belong shouldn't mean we blame ourselves.

Instead, it will be our responsibility to change it, and we will discuss that more in a moment. The problem is we live in a world that no longer prioritises connection.

Perhaps you have noticed many people say they put family first, but they don't act like they do. Think back to Kallie.

Many others say a close community is a great thing and we should have more of it. Yet do they take the time to get to know their neighbours, to prioritise connection?

Do you prioritise social connection, build your tribe and maintain social support?

The bottom line is many of us put close, supportive and caring connections second or last. These priorities result in many of us feeling lonely and socially anxious. We live in western societies that have immersed us in the depths of the fear of social disconnection. It is hardly surprising we have such high levels of social anxiety.

So, don't blame yourself for feeling alone, too different or that you don't have enough, or any, friends. Don't be too concerned that you constantly worry about what everyone says and thinks about you and that you might miss out on what your friends are doing. All these feelings are normal, considering the nature of our society and the times we live in.

Knowing what we are up against socially and despite the barriers in our way, how do we reduce our social anxiety and tame our fears related to people?

Consider the following steps to help you tame your social fears and develop a more significant social connection, even in the age of Covid.

Practical Steps to Tame Social Fears/Anxieties

Step 1. A Strong Sense of Self

We can begin taming our social anxiety by not being so hard on ourselves. Then by building a solid sense of self, we know what we think and feel in our own right, and we are OK with the person we are. We know we are a good person and worthy of others' love, care and support. If you are confident in yourself, you aren't as sensitive to being different. You become less worried about what others say.

It is beyond a book of this type to help teach you to develop a strong sense of self. Though here are a few suggestions to get you on track:

- Write a list of your good qualities. Identify in yourself the positive attributes you would like to see in a friend, to show yourself that you are worthy of friendship and connection. If you can't think of any, ask close friends or family you trust. Sometimes we forget our good qualities, and we need reminding. If you are still struggling, look to the friendship needs we will discuss in a moment and see which of these you meet for others. For example, are you a good listener?
- Ask yourself, if no one knew and I didn't have to answer to anyone, then what do I like? The family might enjoy a good curry but do you, really, or do you like it because they do? Do you like that song because others do? What are your personal preferences?
- Build a connection with nature. We will explore this more in a moment.
- Make more self-time to do what you like, just for you.

Brian liked writing poetry and reading about spirituality and developing a deeper spiritual connection within himself. He said he hadn't done much of it over the last two years but was keen to get back into it. He also liked nature and was excited to re-establish a connection with it.

Another powerful strategy to reduce social anxiety is making people predictable – less scary – so we find it easy to make and maintain connections with them.

How do we make people more predictable and less scary?

One method I like to share is to learn about our basic human needs of friendship. Learn to understand what all of us need to feel safe, secure and satisfied in a social encounter – how to come across to others as a non-threatening friend.

Friendship is becoming a lost art. We make so few close friends these days it can be hard to know what to do to make them, especially if we are used to being alone. Knowing what others need from us to feel friendly and worth being around will make others less intimidating to approach – more predictable. Brian was keen to learn these skills.

Step 2. Know Our Friendship Needs

Being social creatures, we can recognise we all have friendship needs or drives to connect and form supportive groups.

What are our friendship needs or desires?

We can recognise ten friendship needs or basic human desires – we could identify more, but as we shall see, they are all linked. As we start to meet one, we often satisfy many others. Learning to meet ten needs is more straightforward and less complicated than meeting twenty or thirty. Below is a summary of the needs with introductory examples of ways to meet them in others. If you wish to know more about them, I recommend reading my book *The Friendship Key* (Senraan Publishing, Brisbane, 2019).

In essence, we all want the following needs met by everyone we encounter, and they want them met by us. We would meet them differently for different people and different circumstances. For instance, to help our partner feel noticed, we might put our arm around them when we are near them. On the other hand, embracing a work colleague could see us fired and have a sexual harassment suit filed against us.

The following list gives us a general insight into what the brain wants from us to feel comfortable in each other's company.

The aim is to meet these needs in others; it isn't our job to make others meet these needs for us, such as punishing them by not talking to them if they don't seem to care about us. Ultimately, we can only change ourselves. Our primary aim is to meet these friendship needs in others.

Ten Needs of Friendship

1. Valued
We all seek to feel important in some way. We help others feel valued and important by making time for them and being on time. Nothing says you are not worthwhile as a friend – not valued – as much as not making time or always being late. Asking genuinely for someone else's opinions on topics also helps them feel valued.

2. Noticed
How disconnected do you feel if everyone ignores you? Socially, we all seek to be noticed rather than ignored. To help someone feel noticed,

we acknowledge them, preferably by name. Say hi, for instance, as we pass them. If culture permits, look them in the eye, say hello and ask them how they are going. It sounds trivial but is essential.

3. Appreciated

Often, we don't appreciate someone until they aren't there. Feeling appreciated helps us feel we make a critical contribution in their lives. We help others feel appreciated by making them feel indispensable and essential, such as letting them know no one can do what they do the same way they do.

4. Heard

How annoying is it when people don't listen to or hear us or get where we are coming from? We don't want to be around others who don't help us feel heard. We can make someone else feel heard by giving them our undivided attention – no distractions like phones or doing other things at the same time. We can practise active listening, such as nodding to what they say, paraphrasing and saying what we heard back to them, and asking clarifying questions. If you don't know how to apply active listening, it is worth looking it up. A trick, especially for guys in relationships, is don't give the other person advice or a solution unless they specifically ask for it or else you just invalidate them (see below). Always try to show you understand and respect their point of view.

5. Sameness acknowledged

We all like to feel we fit in. One way to do this is to show we are like others, that we have similar views, beliefs and morals. In nature, the enemy is more likely to be different. To help others feel similar, we should look for and acknowledge what we have in common; never focus on differences. By focusing on what we have in common, we tell the other person's brain that we are on their side. A simple way to show we are similar is use small talk, such as 'Looks like it's going to be a hot summer.'

6. Validated/Approved

No one likes to feel they are wrong or stupid, that they can't be themselves. We help others to feel validated and approved by agreeing with them when we can. Don't lie about it, though. Be less critical and judgemental; try to understand more and judge less. We all like others to tell us we are OK as we are.

7. Respected

It goes without saying we all crave and need respect. We specifically help others feel respected by treating them as equals; no one is higher or lower. A powerful way to show respect is to offer others real choices and let them say no without any strange looks or punishment. We never dictate to or order them to do anything. Say more 'please' and 'thank you'. Never impose or force yourself on someone else.

8. Cared For

A good friend is someone we can count on to be there when we are sick and need them most; they care. We help others feel cared for by checking on them to see they are OK. Offer to help others in distress when we can. We should seek support to help us care for others if the burden gets too much.

9. Supported
It might not seem much but receiving support can be life changing. It can give us just the push we need to succeed. Friends are supportive. We can help others feel supported by offering encouragement and assistance without expecting anything in return. Even just words of support and encouragement can go a long way. Especially support someone else's passionate goals if you can.

10. Protected
The bottom line is we all deserve to feel safe. Our friends can be counted on to help us feel safe. We can assist others in feeling safe by speaking up and helping when someone is threatened. Let the law take care of this when needed. No one should feel unsafe.

*****

We are all Friends Here
All someone else's brain wants to know is we are not a threat; we are on their side. The more friendship needs we meet for them, the more their brain recognises this and feels more comfortable around us. The more comfortable they are around us, the less we need to worry about them treating us poorly or acting in a threatening way.

To meet these needs more effectively, we treat others as friends from the beginning. We imagine they are friends or potential friends from the moment we meet them.

If we approach someone as if they are or might be a danger to us, we act as though we aren't their friend, and they will treat us as a threat or enemy in return. Naturally, this will make them and us anxious and a bit afraid of each other.

What if the other person puts us down and makes us feel inferior, like at work or social functions?

We still show them care and respect. We set the standard by treating others the way we hope to be treated. However, we also need to draw the line. Showing respect to others also means respecting ourselves, not taking other people's abuse. Some jobs require us to act subservient, such as serving staff at hotels and functions. It may be that to keep our job, when at work we need to behave as though others are superior. This is a rare compromise. Ideally, we shouldn't have to bow down to anyone just to get along.

Practise your small talk. It's OK not to like it; I don't like it either. Think of small talk as a tool to help others settle down and feel OK around us, a tool to tame each other's social fear.

Especially practise your active listening. The more you listen and validate others, the less you talk and the more they will like you. Most of us love to talk about ourselves or topics we have a passion for. So, see if you can get them to share their passions.

Brian found learning about friendship invaluable. He now had in his mind what to do at work to know he wasn't going to unintentionally come across as awkward or a threat.

Step 3. Build Your Tribe

In a society that doesn't prioritise connection, we can't expect friends will just show up everywhere. If we want social connection, we will have to put in the effort – be proactive. The tribe won't come to us; we have to go to the tribe or, more likely, build our tribe ourselves from scratch.

I know. It sucks, and it shouldn't be this way. But it is.

How can we build a tribe of people we can trust and care for despite the challenges?

Here are some suggestions you can put into practice right now.

Ways to Build a Sense of Tribe Around Us

Make Friendship a Priority

Friendships will only happen if we prioritise them – make them important enough to take the time and put in the effort. Perhaps we need to put friendship higher in our values list we wrote before and in our daily and weekly planner. Plan friendship time with our partner, children, other family members and mates/girlfriends. Don't be disappointed if others don't call us to catch up; be the example they can learn from.

Invite Others Over

Many people are house-proud and worry what others think about their home, so we must be the one to set the trend. Keep the invite and occasion simple – nothing complicated: I've just baked some biscuits, and I'd love to know what you think, for example. Be ready to talk about topics you have in common, not those you see where you differ. If your views on politics are opposite, for instance, then don't talk politics. If you start to disagree and get heated, change the topic or simply agree to disagree. We don't need to agree on everything to still be friends.

I know it gets disheartening when only we make an effort, but these are the times. If we don't persist, often others won't.

Join Common Interest Groups

Go online or to your local community centre and see what hobbies or interest groups you might like to join. For example, I have a lady who found a great sense of friendship in a local knitting group. I have several who joined local hiking, running or cycling groups. Others are learning languages. There may be online social connection sites. I know we have them in my home city, Brisbane.

Create or Join Men-only or Women-only Groups

In tribes, we often had same-sex friends we could relate to and confide in a way we couldn't with the opposite sex. A significant advantage of same-sex friends if we are in a heterosexual relationship is that we can gripe, respectfully, about our partner to our mates/girlfriends and share the burden, not bring the angst home. It is good to have rules for the meetings, such as not speaking poorly of anyone who is not at the meet-up. After all, our aim is to practise meeting friendship needs with everyone, including respect to those not present. I am a big fan of respectful women's circles and men's sheds, for example. They are places where we connect as women and men in more profound, more satisfying ways.

Screen Friends Won't Do

We live such isolated lives these days that we may expect to use social media to meet all our friendship needs and lessen the hollowness. Unfortunately, social media can never meet our friendship needs in a way that truly satisfies us, any more than fans of a celebrity can make them feel genuinely cared for. Most of the time, people on the other side of the screen can't be counted on to be there for us. If you live in Sydney, for instance, the friend in New York isn't going to be there for you after a horrible breakup, giving you a hug or offering a spare bed. We need real, local friends in our tribe.

* * * * *

A teacher I shared friendship ideas with took creating a local tribe far further than I expected. She loved the tribal idea so much – and recognised how critical it was for her – that she made a pendant for each member of her 'tribe' to wear. The pendant bore the names of all her tribe's members. She also created a set of respectful guiding rules and principles, framed them and shared them among the group, and arranged regular meetings and other ways of supporting each other. I was duly impressed. She felt much better for it, and I am told her friends in the tribe did too.

Common What Ifs

What If I Feel Unworthy of Other People's Friendship?

Like Brian, it isn't uncommon to have suffered traumas in our past. These horrible experiences can negatively impact the story we have of ourselves. Remember, how we feel is mainly determined by our story, the dream we live by. The trauma, for instance, might convince us we are a terrible person or unlovable or not worthwhile. This is our natural reaction. Besides, if we weren't any of these negative things, why didn't people care for and protect us and help us feel we belonged and fitted in. In essence, our past traumas create stories about us in our minds that prevent us from meeting and keeping friends. We will introduce ways to rewrite such traumas in a later section. Suffice to say, we all deserve to be cared for, respected and supported. We all deserve the warmth and safety of close friends.

What If I'm So Scared that I Can't Leave the House?

Start slowly. Only invite over people you are comfortable with. Go with them to the footpath then the street. Practise the calming meditations we learned earlier. By being calm in a particular place we create a calming memory of it, making it less scary next time. Gradually, leave the house and go further and further, stop, practise feeling calm, then come home. This process is called desensitisation. We will discuss it more soon.

What If I'm Scared of Catching Something Fatal From Someone Else?
In the time of Covid, this can be a reasonable worry. We will look at ways to resolve Covid-related fears in a coming chapter.

Those who Matter don't Mind

To be honest, the ultimate and best cure for social anxiety and fear would be once again to have close and supportive communities and families. Unfortunately, we don't always have those.

After discussing fear and how we should face it, Brian and I looked at his worst fear. We used some of the steps we will soon learn to overcome individual fears. His worse fear was making a fool of himself around others. I asked him, 'Do you suddenly stop wanting to be close friends with some of your best friends or people close to you because they made a fool of themselves once or twice in front of you?' 'No,' he said, 'of course not.' 'So, would your friends – your true and trusted friends – think any less of you if you made a fool of yourself in front of them, if they are true friends?' He stopped a moment, and soon it looked like a lightbulb moment of realisation. He said, 'I guess not if they're my real friends.' We continued another tack.

'How many people in the supermarket are you likely to ever meet again or get to know well?' 'Well, none of them,' he replied. 'So, you are telling me you are worried about what people think of you although you will never be close friends with them or likely meet them again?' 'I guess I am,' he replied.

'So, what you are saying [he paraphrased without me prompting him] is if I make a fool of myself in front of the people that matter most, it doesn't matter; they will still accept me. And if I make a fool of myself among people I don't know, it doesn't matter since I won't have anything to do with them, and it won't affect my life anyway.' I nodded. 'Yep.'

The following week I saw Brian again. He said almost all his social anxiety had left him. He showed it by letting me know he wore a shabby shirt he would normally never wear in public because he'd be too self-conscious. He let me know he was pretty OK to leave the house now and go shopping. Typically, I find it takes longer for such fears to settle, but it was relatively quick in this case.

Was he ready to go back to work yet? That took a few more weeks.

* * * *

PANIC DISORDER

It is worth pointing out here that one of the greatest fears people with panic disorder have is that it will happen in public. They worry so much they will have a panic attack in public that they do have one. As was true for Brian, if we suffer from panic disorder it is helpful to change our perspective. For instance, if we saw someone having a panic attack in public, would we think any less of them? Probably not. So why would they think any less of us? Besides, how many who see us have a panic attack will we see again? And, as Brian realised, if they are our friends, they won't judge us for it. They will more than likely want to help. If they aren't our friends and we never see them again, does it really matter?

> This process of seeing from different perspectives is called reframing. We will discuss this more soon.

Now let us look at how to reduce fears from the media. Does what you see in the media scare you?

CHAPTER 8

BEWARE THE NEWS!

Stage 6. Dial Down the Scary Stuff

I'd known Leo for over ten years. He was a regular. In his youth, Leo had the unfortunate experience of being shot and barely surviving an unprovoked assault. Then, upon arriving in Australia over twenty years ago and looking more foreign than most, he suffered blatant racial prejudice. Leo said he never felt he fitted in, though he tried. Leo's army-style cropped hairstyle and bulging midriff gave no hint that he was an intelligent guy. Unfortunately, his bouts of depression and PTSD left him unable to work. He was on a pension and would find part-time work where he could. He had a few friends he visited sparingly but mainly was a private chap. Since I'd known him, he'd been friendly, polite, forthright, honest and kind. He cared for the wellbeing of others. He would never even think of using or mistreating anyone. However, once Covid struck, I noticed a disturbing change.

Since Leo was without much to do, he watched a lot of news, especially from the western European country that spoke his native tongue. When he saw stories of immigrants robbing or bashing people in Australia, he became outraged. When he heard Australia was letting in refugees from Middle Eastern countries, he clenched his fist. He raised his voice, 'Are the politicians crazy letting murderers and criminals into this country?' When the topic of people from India came up, 'Don't trust them,' he said. 'They are only after one thing. They don't respect life as we do.' Slowly, he showed signs of intolerance, anger and aggression I'd never seen in such a gentle soul before. Then came the distrust.

'Princess Diana is alive,' he told me. 'She faked her death. It was the only way to stop the press from hounding her.' 'The government brought the twin towers down; no buildings collapse like that, even after an impact. Besides, he said, the government knows who comes and goes into the country. They knew what was happening all along.' He claimed that the Covid virus was made in a laboratory to f**k the black people and immigrants. 'Treatments for Covid? Don't tell me the government doesn't have treatments they are keeping for themselves. And have you noticed only in the US are they freezing people?' He noticed in New York, for instance, that bodies were being stored in mobile freezers since their morgues were full. 'What better way to take the virus and modify it later to kill even more people? One and one make two,' he said definitively. 'I'm not stupid!'

The effects of fear can present in many ways, like generalised anxiety or tension where we are constantly on alert for some impending doom. They can show up as trying to avoid places and situations where we fear for our life. Perhaps it will present as a lack of sleep, poor concentration or keeping busy so we don't have time to think, or as completely shutting off and emotionally disconnecting us from our feelings – emotional detachment. In Leo's case, the fears he felt that related to Covid happened to manifest as anger, aggression, intolerance, paranoia and distrust.

Leo's fear was completely understandable. The media had been saturating us with everything Covid, focusing on death, telling us it will all get worse. It was made to sound like the end of the world, and we could die at any moment. If we don't have other people we trust to check if we are thinking reasonably, it's easy to get lost down a rabbit hole of fear and distrust. Leo lacked the opportunity to have a clear discussion and consider the facts from different perspectives. He wasn't the only one. We'll touch on another extreme case in Chapter 17.

Do you know anyone who has become so scared by the news they are gripped by horrible fears of conspiracies and paranoia? It is all terribly distressing. I wouldn't wish it on anyone.

We live in an era unlike any in history. For the first time, the news is available twenty-four seven. It used to be we'd have to wait for the evening news on TV, or the daily paper in the morning, or hourly broadcasts on the radio. Not anymore; now we have live feeds as it's happening, and it is so accessible we can check it on our phones anytime we like. In addition, we have social media, with people offering opinions and theories without any foundation in fact. Of course, this further feeds our fears and paranoia: yes, the government is against us, and so are the doctors; I thought so!

Leo was subject to preferencing media that was significantly raising his fear burden. What about the media and your fear burden? How much is the media contributing to your level of daily fear? Consider some of the following examples and see if this is how the media is contributing to your anxiety. Once we know what we are up against, we can work on ways to counter it.

Four Common Media Fears

Fear of Missing Vital Updates

How many times do you check the news in a day? Be honest. What drives us to keep pulling out our phones, or look at our computer or TV to check what's happening in the world? I mean, during the recent Covid outbreak, it made sense to keep a look out for updates and changes to restrictions. But we can look at the news so much that the sheer volume can overwhelm us; it can be too much to take in. Worse, with so much new information spread on social media almost instantly, it can leave us feeling like we are constantly out of touch and behind: So why am I the last in my group of friends to know? Why am I so behind compared to everyone else?

Readily available news should bring us comfort. It lets us know nothing around us is threatening, that there is nothing to worry about. It adds information to make our world more predictable, so our brain can settle knowing it doesn't need a plan; if there is no threat, there is nothing to fear. Instead, the way our media works today, so much information is available we can't process it all. What we don't understand makes us afraid. And we haven't even mentioned the stories the news focuses on that are told to make us fearful on purpose. More on that in a moment.

Then we can be afraid to get behind: what am I missing that is important? And if we don't know the news our friends or family do, we have the added fear of being out of the loop. We become afraid of getting behind, out of touch, and being judged for it: What, you don't know that? You're kidding, right?

But to keep up to date with so much information is time-consuming. It can take hours just to filter through some of it.

The scramble to be informed can then see us quickly get behind in other parts of our life. We spend too much time looking at media. Then, the next thing we know, we don't have time to get everything done. Like Kallie earlier, we fear there is too much to do and not enough hours in the day.

As a simple exercise to see how much time news takes up in your day, use the back of your worry book. I'm sure you have one by now, right? Now, every time you look at a screen to find out anything – not for phone calls or to play games – write it down. Then, tally up the times at the end of the day and week. Some phones have an app that shows your screen use too. How many hours was it? Does this amount of time surprise you?

Now, how would you feel if you didn't look at the news for seven consecutive days? Does that bring on feelings of dread or discomfort? If so, perhaps fear of missing news plays a significant role in your life.

Fear from Is It True?

Our fear from media gets worse when we learn that much of the information may not be entirely accurate or is misleading. This isn't just the age of information overload and news 24/7; it is also the era when a fact is not a fact. In recent years we have seen media representatives say their facts are different. For example, the so called 'alternative facts' described by President Donald Trump's counsellor, Kellyanne Conway, in 2017. If a fact isn't even a recognisable fact or truth anymore, how are we supposed to know what or whom to believe?

Then we learn that the modern media is being manipulated for politics, money and power; there are reasons many out there are manipulating information. We can be lied to and not know it. We can be driven to believe falsehoods that seem genuine. The very heart of truth we hold onto can come into question.

No wonder Leo was struggling to make sense of what he was seeing in the media; how much of it was true?

When our brain doesn't have any facts or truths to hold onto, the world suddenly becomes uncertain. An uncertain world is an unfamiliar and unpredictable world. The unpredictability creates a fear response, as we have already noted.

How much of what you learn from the media do you trust? How much of it isn't true? Not knowing fact from fiction in an environment where we are overloaded with information is bound to add further to our fear burden.

Fear from Factionalised News

The average human response to being afraid is to search for our tribe. As we've seen, we are made to feel safe and secure among others like us, among kin. When it comes to news and media, we search out those with similar views, opinions, beliefs and fears. The next thing we know, we have opposing factions at each other's throats and fear levels escalating. We become afraid of others who vehemently disagree with us. Some exchanges can come close to blows.

Have you felt scared lately during a heated disagreement?

Consider politics as an example. Social media has made it evident that the people with more liberal or left-leaning political views will follow left-leaning, liberal news. They will search out and find left-leaning information sites and sources. Similarly, people with more conservative, right-wing, nationalistic views or beliefs will follow right-leaning and conservative news. They will search out and find right-leaning information sites and sources, such as Sky and

Fox News. This essentially divides the people in communities into opposing factions: the left and the right. Both sides are convinced they are correct and virtuous.

In addition, we find people in echo chambers of news and social media – places where views are echoed among like-minded folk. These echo chambers – Facebook and Twitter are just two examples – breed extremist views. This is primarily thanks to the people in them no longer considering alternative ways of seeing things. As we noted from the needs of friendship, we all seek to be validated and approved. In a society already afraid – for reasons we mentioned earlier – we can expect people to polarise into extremist and intolerant opposing groups.

But the more we divide ourselves into factions, the more we highlight and focus on our differences. As we now know, focusing on differences makes us appear like enemies to each other. Moreover, a focus on difference breeds fear. Factionalised and opposing news media has heightened the fear in our society. We even become afraid of our neighbours. Are they from the left or the right?

Do you feel safer in a society where there are people who have passionate opposite views to yours and are prepared to physically fight to defend their faction's beliefs?

Fear to Gain Our Attention

Perhaps you've noticed private media peddles fear like lollies to hungry children. The news media knows that emotional stories sell – they get people watching and listening. The primary emotion they use to get our attention, particularly when it comes to news, is fear.

How many stories of murders, wars, killings, gun deaths, disease outbreaks, gangs roaming the streets, violent crime and hostile immigrants keep showing up in the news? How many stories on violence has your media source shown in the last twenty-four hours; another mass shooting, perhaps? It is as though the media is making us look by offering the most powerful and disgusting, fearful stories they can find. And they are doing it on purpose.

Fear sells. It makes us look because our brain is wired to prioritise fear. If we don't make the scary our top priority, we could die by not planning for a threat. So, the media can sell advertising by you and me taking the bait and looking at its gruesome news. Fear makes a profit; fear is big bucks.

Of course, if all we see on the news is violence and fear-inducing stuff, our brain can come to believe we don't live in a very safe neighbourhood or a safe world. Soon we can be afraid of – and show hostility, intolerance and aggression towards – people who are different from us, just as Leo did. The media has made us into enemies and potential enemies. It could have focused on our similarities, our shared humanity but, instead, it consciously chose not to. No wonder we are afraid of our neighbours, are intolerant and struggle to create united and supportive communities. We have been trained to be too scared to; it's dangerous out there!

It would be tough to quantify just how much fear the media adds to our life, our neighbourhoods and between countries. But, considering how much influence media has in determining our stories and dreams about the world, we can reasonably assume the fear burden they add is substantial. Who has the media taught you to be afraid of?

So, how do we reduce the fear burden of news and media? Here are some recommendations.

Reduce the Fear Burden of News and Media

Remember: Less is More

Stop looking! Seriously! It makes sense that if the news makes us fearful, anxious or scared, then we cut back on watching it.

How much should we cut back?

That is up to you. How much do you think you need to? I recommend looking at the news once a day for less than an hour. It's a good beginning.

But what about our fear of missing something important, not being in the loop?

If we have more face-to-face social connections, we will automatically know what is relevant and vital. This is crucial: at no time should we feel deficient because we miss something in the media. Besides, I'm sure one of us will know at least a little news worth knowing to share with the rest. It also goes without saying we should never make fun of someone who doesn't know the news we do.

If you are serious about wanting to detox from the media's fear, try not looking at it for two weeks. Unless, of course, your work demands you keep up with current events. When I was on my sabbatical in my early twenties, I spent weeks to months not looking at the news. And guess what? The world was still here.

Be Selective

Seek a news source that is less likely to spin the news and is more reliable. Avoid sources that promote fear, conspiracies, anger, intolerance and hate. You know the ones. Don't let them sucker you in so they can make a buck at your expense.

And don't use social media sites for news, especially places that only show one side. As we have seen, news echo chambers may make us feel less anxious knowing about others like us but, in the end, that also makes many more potential enemies for us. It highlights those who are different and ultimately makes us more afraid. Making sure we see opposing sides to a story allows us to share information as respected individuals who aren't each other's enemy. We may interpret the data differently, but we also have more information to agree on and bring us together. It allows us to be less factionalised and scared because of it.

Multisource

If you want to know about a topic, try to find at least three opposing views on the topic. Don't just stick with one source. If there is a truth, it is somewhere between the facts and opinions we have read. Try to keep an open mind. If we go in with a firm view before starting, we will search and find what we want or need to. The process of finding information or data that will confirm an opinion we already have is called confirmation bias. Social media echo chambers are full of confirmation bias: people seeing what they want or need to see, not anything resembling truth.

Try to research knowing your bias and finding information beyond it – opposing views that disprove you.

Personally, I learned a long time ago to always keep an open mind; after all, I might be wrong. That way, I know I'm open to seeing more facts and better able to see what is actually happening.

Connect with Community

Talk with others in an open way that allows sharing of information among open minds. The aim of social meetings should be more about listening and validating, trying to understand each other's points of view. Focus on what you agree on first. As we've seen, we are more likely to listen to friends than enemies. Once we agree, we then share what we know with respect for those with different opinions who have seen additional information or have different experiences.

This is a great way to have a respectful discussion with anyone. First, we find common ground to agree on. Then we add our ten cents worth. Then we explore why we each see it differently. For example, ask 'What did you see that I didn't?' and vice versa?

The aim is not to win: I'm right; you must believe what I do. The objective is to share information and accept we may both be wrong and probably are. After all, we can't truly know we are correct until we have all the information, not just a tiny bit of it.

The key, once again, is to keep an open mind, to not let fear restrict what we see. If we share what we saw, read or learned, then the rest of us can see it too and discuss it freely and see where we agree.

Apolitical community discussion forums or meetings would be ideal. Obviously, it would need a flexible and robust moderator. Do any places or people come to mind?

Unfortunately, Leo did not speak to others with many different opinions. Instead, his fear led him to form very self-righteous views; he had to be correct. Soon he believed so-called facts and theories although they were transparent lies.

Hold Media Accountable

In the USA, before the 1980s, they had fair media rules. The rules required each major media outlet to provide equal time for opposing views or takes on important topics. Then the fair media laws were dropped, and there was a free for all; the media could focus on what sells rather than what informs. Now, in the USA and many other countries we have factionalised and sensational news driven by profit no matter the social and personal consequences.

Is this the type of media we want, peddling fear and dividing us? Should we want to, how can we change it?

We vote. Democracy allows us, the people, to change laws. If our representatives don't do what we need them to do, we vote them out and replace them with someone with like-minded views.

Let's be clear. We are not suggesting stopping freedom of the press in order to hold our governments accountable. On the contrary, the fundamentals of freedom of the press to hold governments to account and prevent the darkness of ignorance can and should remain for a healthy democracy to thrive. We are simply recommending laws that ensure the media informs more than it causes unnecessary distress – media that focuses on our similarities more than our differences and cares about the wellbeing of the people, so they feel safe and secure.

Sound like a fairy tale?

My niece visited Japan several years ago. She said the news there was much calmer than in Australia, less sensationalised, less shocking and less scary yet still very informative. Their media is still privately owned. A significant difference is they still have fair media laws.

*****

The bottom line: if the media makes us feel uncomfortable, anxious or unwell, switch it off. Don't look or listen. Better still, perhaps try to change our media through insisting on fair media laws?

For many of us, the fear generated by our media is a substantial burden. It doesn't have to be.

* * * * *

Leo still grapples with the fears of Covid and having the vaccine. He is vaccinated. He did cut back on watching the news. He recognised it was making him upset. He still lives a mostly isolated life. Despite great encouragement, he doesn't want to make new friends. We keep in regular touch.

* * * * *

It is difficult for many of us to realise just how much fear is lurking in the background – how enormous our fear burden is. It is like a bad smell; we don't notice it after a while. But that doesn't mean the fear isn't adversely impacting us. It also doesn't mean we can't live calmer lives.

A powerful resource and skill that can remove us from many of the fears associated with modern life is nature. We may not be the outdoors type. That's OK. Nature is an excellent fear-taming resource for everyone. We will learn how to tap into nature as a fear taming skill in the next chapter.

CHAPTER 9

NATURE HELPS

Stage 7. Tap into Nature's Peace

Do you have a place in a garden, on a beach, in a forest, or by a creek that offers your soul a sense of rest and inner contentment, a welcoming break from the rigours of your daily grind?

Nature can be the answer to many of our mental struggles if we choose to connect with it.

It's Only Natural!

The air was crisp and fresh; there was no light but for the brilliance of a soup of stars painted across the cloudless sky above me. Crickets chirped. The odd cow mooed in the distance as I trod the loose gravel of the country road not far from my parent's farm. It was semester break from uni, a time I'd spend recovering down on my parent's hobby farm in southern New South Wales; on less than three hundred acres, they ran some cattle and sheep. After dinner, I went for a walk, as I often did, to a spot that was less than five hundred metres from the house. It was past the farm gate and down the road towards a dip where there were a dozen or more old gum – eucalypt – trees on either side. I found my favourite tree, sat, and connected.

I had two favoured spots to sit quietly on the farm. One was about a third the way up a hill at the back of the property. The view was for miles out across the countryside, which was mostly flat with just a few more hills to the left. Not far below me was a large dam, more prominent than an Olympic-sized swimming pool, cut into the side of the slope. My attention was rarely on the dirty water of the dam, the cows below, the small farmhouse, or the hay or machinery sheds. Instead, it focused on the vast land as flat as a carpet spotted with trees. The other favoured place was sitting under the old gum tree past the farm gate. It felt right.

Have you ever sat beside someone quietly, both of you still, and felt a connection with them that transcended words? There was a feeling about them that felt right? That is somewhat what it was like under this tree for me. Within months of my parents moving to the farm from town when I was still finishing high school, I'd discovered it. Its branches weren't spread out flat and sprouted outwards like others; they were primarily vertical. The trunk, covered in flaking, peeling bark, was too big for me to put my arms around even if I wanted to. The spot was away from the road, near a fence, and best of all, it had a nice place to sit that wasn't near an ant nest. I spent hours there during my breaks meditating, contemplating and just sitting. It helped me develop a connection with myself and the tree, beyond what I term Land and Indigenous Australians call Country.

To sit under this wise and ancient being – as I came to know it – was to bring peace. Gone was the busyness of life, study and expectation. Gone were the worries about being accepted. Here I could sit and feel life differently. Contemplating the nature of the tree imagining what it might feel like as a tree on Country was immensely enlightening.

Contemplating the tree, I would often ask questions to better reflect on it in different ways. For example, what would this tree feel or notice? Would it notice the insect scurrying over it? Probably not. Would it notice the rumble of cars and trucks nearby? Most likely. Would it notice me? Trees sense and react to their world too. What would it be like to feel and sense as a tree? Could it feel Country? To contemplate the tree was to feel Country – the Land.

To empathise with this tree was also a way to slow down a hurried and disconnected soul.

Does your life feel hurried? Does your inner being feel disconnected, lonely, lacking a greater sense of self and being, a greater understanding of place and purpose?

You are not alone.

For eons, human beings have lived closely with the natural world – nature. We were part of nature, and nature was part of us. Nature gave us a sense of belonging, a sense of peace. It also allowed us to develop a more resilient and confident sense of self when returning to others' company. This is only a glimmer of what connecting with nature and this tree offered me.

Although connecting with nature and realising the benefits goes back beyond history, using nature as a therapeutic tool to assist with mental health, such as anxiety, is relatively recent. Today it is termed eco-therapy.

Eco-therapy essentially means connecting with nature. It can be achieved from nature retreats, hiking in forests, sitting under a tree, camping in the wild, or tending to a garden or pot plants at home.

Nature, by and large, is calming and soothing. So long as there are no immediate threats like bears, lions or wolves, being in and experiencing nature takes us to a whole different – chill-out – level, as I found it did for me.

The property of nature I find most beneficial for reducing our fear burden is it slows us down.

Nature Slows Us

Learning the secret of fear earlier has taught us that our body uses fear to increase our strength and speed – how fast we react. We perceive time differently when afraid. It is as though fear takes us into a different time zone, which seems slower somehow. For example, people have described objects like an arrow coming towards them in slow motion. Another example is fighter pilots as they flick their nimble planes through narrow canyons. They are running on adrenaline – fear – the whole time to react the fastest possible. Their heart rates can reach peaks well beyond those during regular flying. In a busy life, we can know this speeding up effect of fear as being hyped up, buzzing with energy, until the adrenalin wears off and we fall asleep.

Our modern lives can often speed us up, using fear to do it. By contrast, nature slows us down.

Have you ever noticed how fast life is in a city compared to the speed and pace of life in a forest or bushland? In the city, it is go-go-go; time is money, no time to waste, I have tasks to do, people to see, family to care for, bills to pay. If only I had more time! Does this remind you of Kallie and Belinda, earlier? Contrast this to being in nature and on Country.

Does a tree care whether we show up? No. Do the birds hurry us along? No. Do the bees always travel at warp speed? No. Does a stream rush to get to the sea? No. Nature, by and large, runs at a much slower pace. Be in nature long enough, and we become part of its slower time zone; we tune into it. Nature innately chills us out. It does the opposite of fear.

One of the questions I would regularly ask patients with mental illness is, do they like spending time in the countryside? Many city-folk who have spent their whole lives among buildings and houses aren't comfortable being in nature, which is OK. However, living in a city like Brisbane, where bushland and beaches are close by, it isn't uncommon to find people drawn to nature. Some grew up camping, fishing and surfing. Like me, others grew up in the country proper on a farm. Many, like Brian, earlier, who are anxious and struggling to cope have lost the connection to nature they now realise was beneficial.

Consider other examples.

Take Mandy, late twenties. She is on a working visa from Canada in a job she hates with a tyrannical boss. Back in Canada, she'd be hiking regularly alone or with friends. She loved the feel of the great outdoors – its peace and quiet. She worked long hours and rushed most of her day. Mandy took to reconnecting with nature like a pro. Through hiking, mountain climbing and just sitting among the beauty of the natural world around her, she found it much easier to calm down. We dealt with her fear of her boss later. Within weeks she felt back to her old self.

Then there is Josh, newly married, mid-twenties, working in IT, and so stressed out of his brain he can't get a sense of peace no matter what he does. We tried medication without success; he desperately wanted to give them a try. He indeed needed a holiday to reset his mind and mental rest. The two weeks of medical leave made a significant impact, especially him using the time to go to the beach and walk in nearby parks and bushland. He grew up near the beach and, in his youth, his father would take him camping. It wasn't a long break, but he was back to full-time work and coping much better. He maintained his regular bushwalks and visits to the ocean. He fully admits connection with nature is an invaluable strategy he is more than willing to keep.

Then there is Jess, in her late forties, on a journey of self-discovery, working in education. She often finds her mind a jumble and readily overcommits herself to helping too many people and being involved with too much. What helps her enormously is she begins her day with grounding – literally her bare feet touching the earth. She also meditates and finds walks in nature amazingly soothing. She lives opposite parkland and visits it every day.

I know elderly couples who find peace in their garden; they can be there all day long. I know several young men and women who find surfing is their thing – like the Hemsworth brothers, who as well as acting also apparently like riding their boards on waves. They just happen to live a few hundred kilometres down the road in Byron Bay. Chris, you will recall, is famous for playing Thor, the god of thunder in movies.

When I walk by the beach, especially in the morning or late evenings, many people are out taking in the sea breeze and soothing vista. Most are walking. Many are sitting, their eyes focused yonder.

What eco-therapy recommendations would I suggest to help reduce your fear burden? Consider the following:

- Look to your past and see what connection with nature in childhood holds the best memories for you. For me, it was on the farm. Then find places like it that remind you of those feelings, places where you feel you can connect with it.

- Prioritise time in nature. Put it in your weekly planner. It won't happen if you don't see it as essential and make the time.
- If you aren't sure what to do, write a list of options with pros and cons. Do you like hiking? Do you like walking on a beach? Is there a nearby beach? Do you enjoy sitting under a tree or meditating in a park and know such a place where you can feel safe? Perhaps you like tending plants; we don't need a garden to care for our cellulose friends.
- When in nature, let it take you into its time zone, notice how it runs slower and feel yourself fitting into it.
- If you are willing, contemplate the nature around you; imagine what might be noticed by a tree or by a crow or an insect. It's probably not so settling to watch and consider a busy Willie Wagtail; they can be more jittery and on edge than us!

Our brain has the extraordinary ability to put itself into the shoes of someone or something else. As a result, it can help us reconnect with a calmer, more natural state of being than we may be used to.

Why not see how you can use nature to slow and tame your fears.

Before we finish using eco-therapy as a fear-reducing tool, it is worth remembering nature offers us another essential way to tame our fear burden: it can help reduce the enormous power of status anxiety.

Nature as a Balm for Status Anxiety

Oh, no. Am I wearing the right brand of shoes, clothes or makeup? Is my car more expensive and more prominent than theirs? I bet I can earn more than them!

Keeping up with the Joneses can be very stressful. It is also very common – so common and popular that they made a TV show based on it. We see a family having to keep up with the richest and best-looking people. You know the family I'm talking about. Daily we are constantly reminded of what we don't have and others do. We are made to feel inferior and different. These feelings of being, and having, less than others create intense anxieties – fears – that dominate our lives. When we judge ourselves on what we own and how important we need to be, we set ourselves up for status anxiety.

Status anxiety is a fear fuelled primarily by us not feeling important enough in our society – not having enough wealth or being sufficiently influential in others' eyes. How many people have you met who are driven to have the bigger house in the wealthier suburb, the most prestigious car, and need to talk about their expensive and exclusive holidays?

When they drop off their children at school – especially private schools – I have mums tell me that they are eyeing off how expensive each other's cars are, what designer clothes each of them is wearing, their shoes, hair and makeup. Those poor stressed mothers have quite a reputation to maintain thanks to status anxiety. Of course, choosing to be caught up in the status anxiety merry-go-round is a personal choice. Ultimately, if you want to feel this added level of fear/stress, it is up to you.

But why do we do it? Why are we trying to have what others have? Why do we feel like we need to be important and 'better' in other people's eyes to the point where it leaves us feeling anxious if we're not? We can find answers in the 10 needs of friendship we briefly looked at earlier.

Some of the friendship needs that help us form supportive, safe tribal groups are our desire to feel similar to others and be valued and appreciated. In other words, we like to feel invaluable, have influence and not be too different from everyone else. If we don't meet these desires, then we feel anxious, afraid. The fear is nature telling us we need to satisfy these desires to feel safe and survive.

So, if we don't own the same car, clothes or mobile phone as those around us who we want to fit in with, we feel anxious because we feel different. Suppose we have a smaller house, cheaper car or less prestigious job. In that case, we can feel anxiety because we think we are of lesser importance. Then if we think we aren't doing a job that is recognised as essential and has influence or power, we can feel unappreciated. Some of us find it hard to feel appreciated if we do a job we think anyone can do.

Status anxiety is real and affects more of us than we might admit. Thankfully, status anxiety has a potential antidote if we are prepared to use nature.

For starters, nature allows us a calmer state of mind, a more peaceful way of viewing the world and ourselves. For example, nature cares nothing about our social standing. A tree, bird or fish doesn't treat us differently according to our job, how many houses we own, or what car we drive or are driven in. And can we really expect a mosquito to bite a billionaire or politician any less than, say, a sanitation worker, assuming they all aren't wearing repellent?

To be in nature, especially to spend time on Country, offers us the chance to relieve ourselves of many social fears by helping us see ourselves in a different light, away from social norms and expectations, even if it is only temporary. It offers us a way of seeing ourselves that is more accepting. Nature doesn't discriminate.

Nature also offers the soothing hope of reminding us we are part of something greater than ourselves we can connect with. It provides us with a sense of home and belonging. Nature reminds us we are human beings in our own right, worthy of the same respect and care as any creature or living thing in the natural world. We are an essential part of a larger whole we can connect with and feel part of. We are all creations of nature and part of it.

How do we connect with nature to reduce our social anxieties?

We can begin by following the earlier recommendation of how to use eco-therapy.

Coming to the city from the country was quite a culture shock. First, I went from a town where we greeted each other on the street. We lifted a finger as a wave when we passed each other on country roads. Then I arrived in a city where we avoided eye contact, mainly focusing on getting to where we needed to be. The city, for me, was a place filled with lots of people, but they were disconnected. They barely knew each other and were constantly in judgement. When I started uni, the first question I was asked was what school I went to. The second question was what suburb I lived in or grew up in. The third inevitable question was what my parents did for a living. The city was terribly lonely, and not just for me. There was loneliness all around and high anxiety levels. But what made it hardest of all was a lack of Country.

I think I watched The Man from Snowy River movie over ten times when it came out while I was trapped in Sydney with my studies. It reminded me of the country I knew from my youth. I played a cassette of the soundtrack until it wore out. Weekend bushwalks in Ku-ring-gai Chase National Park were my adopted saviour. They helped me get through some difficult times. Eventually, my parents sold the farm to be near my sister's children here in Queensland. However, the country down south and around where I grew up still holds a powerful and special place inside me.

*****

I know nature and connecting with it isn't everyone's cup of tea. Still, suppose we want to reduce our fear burden, especially our social anxieties and expectations. In that case, it can be an excellent resource. All we need to do is take the time and connect.

*****

How did Kallie reduce her fear burden and find greater peace from her anxieties of regret? How many of the above strategies did she find helpful?

Kallie came in after a few sessions much calmer and seemed more settled in herself. 'I know what I need to do,' she told me. 'Thank you,' she said. I asked her what made the difference?

She said that talking about achieving a balance of self – from the Balance of Self Model mentioned earlier – played a part. So did the Balance for Parents, to know the needs within the family. But what helped her most of all was the homework of making a priority list.

Writing that list and sharing it with her husband finally helped her realise what she needed to do. She loved her job immensely and didn't want to threaten it, but she also knew she was giving it much more time than she needed to. No more late nights and early starts, no more saying yes to everyone and taking on whatever they asked. Now she realised she needed to set limits. Gone were the regrets that she'd miss out connecting with her children and look back wishing it was different. This was the right balance for her.

What other strategies did Kallie use to reduce her fear burden?

Surprisingly, considering her workload, she said she already knew how to compartmentalise. She found it easy to separate work and life.

She wasn't interested in mindfulness. Instead, she had decided to start yoga again, having enjoyed it in the past.

The household was already orderly, with structure and routines well set in place over many years. And the kids seemed to be doing fine. There were no signs of stress, and they had access to their father if Kallie wasn't around.

Taking on fear from the media?

What media? Kallie knew how to keep well informed with facts. She needed them in her job. She chose to waste no time on social media and the innuendo of echo chambers.

Did she spend time in nature?

Their family enjoyed the beach and had plenty of beaches to choose from.

What about slowing down from her busy schedule?

Kallie felt these were enough changes for now, and that was OK.

But did she want to work on past fears and eliminate them?

Why? She'd found what she was after and was ready to dive into her life as a calmer, more focused self.

The fear burden for each of us is going to be different. Your level might be higher or lower or different from mine, your partners, or your friends and neighbours. And that is how it should be. Each of us is different and, like Kallie, we often have the choice as to how much fear or stress we are prepared to accept in our life. Suppose Kallie ever wanted to resolve individual fears, like those of her childhood. In that case, I'd probably recommend she work on reducing her fear burden more if she was willing. But with her life so organised, I suspect there wouldn't be too many areas to work to reduce.

* * * * *

What we have just shared are but a few ways to reduce our fear burden in our life. There are many others not mentioned here that you might wish to explore further. Some are to lessen the fear burden for you and some are to reduce fears more broadly. Consider the following suggestions if you are searching to reduce your fear burden further:

- Learn to teach yoga, tai chi or pilates.
- Help support retreats for people to learn fear-taming skills.
- Join a woman's circle of supportive, non-judgemental, respectful women, or the equivalent for men.
- Engage in groups – or start one – focused on reclaiming local forests, streams and parks. We have several here in Brisbane.
- Connect with indigenous cultures still practising traditional ways to help you develop a deeper spiritual connection to Country.
- Offer support to families with young children. They often need it.
- Be active in the community. Help your neighbours, especially if they struggle. The more supported we feel, the less we fear.

Just as there is a massive fear burden out there – if we look, we can find it at every turn – so there are many ways to reduce it.

* * * * *

How did you go with your list of fears from earlier? Have any of them now been resolved? For instance, if social anxiety was part of your main fear, has that already been reduced or been resolved, like it was for Brian? Has slowing your busy life allowed you to solve problems and reduce fears you just haven't had time to before? Has cutting back on media and spending more time in nature allowed you to chill?

Now that our fear burden is lessened, we are better positioned to resolve any remaining individual fears.

How do we tame our individual fears, such as fear of losing our job, our partner leaving, contracting a severe illness, or dying?

We use the secrets of understanding fear we learned earlier to guide us.

PART 2
FROM FEAR MONSTER TO FRIEND

Melinda was an emotional wreck, though you might struggle to find a reason why. She had a lovely, well-behaved one-year-old child and the complete and unwavering support of a calm husband who was doing whatever he could to help. She had a job in the health industry and was very good at it. She loved her job. Melinda was a healthy, slim, fit-looking woman in her mid to late twenties.

What bothered her terribly were severe panic attacks – fear maxed out – at least several times a day. These terrible episodes would leave her a trembling mess and unable to do even the simplest tasks. She'd had to take weeks off work and was worried she might never be well enough to go back. The day I first saw her, Melinda was particularly distressed. She'd seen numerous doctors over many months, been admitted to hospital more than once, and been on many medications, but was still getting worse. Tears flowed. Her hands covered her face. She didn't want to leave her beautiful daughter without a mother.

Thankfully, by the end of her second appointment and our discussion about fear – talking about many of the secrets of fear we learned earlier – she had already started to notice relief. She told me she began to feel hope. We worked on mindfulness skills – the ones we described in Chapter 4 – and breathing exercises to stop her acute panic attacks, or at least settle them when they showed up. I recommended regular walks, and she found some benefit. Then we tackled her worst fears – her fear list – one by one.

Our road to recovery isn't always fast or smooth, and this was the case for Melinda. Often, she'd tell me she was feeling worse again, then feel better after she left the session, at least for several days. Each time she came back, we'd focus on the fear that bothered her most at that time – the worst case running through her head – and work to resolve it.

Within six weeks, she felt much better. Sudden episodes of fear were infrequent. She practised her skills to resolve and tame her fears, keeping her fear burden low.

Within a few months, Melinda wanted to come off her medication. She was back at work. Only very occasionally would a fear come up, and she'd be on it and taming it before it got out of hand.

She was expecting another child a year later and was thrilled about it. This was despite two of her greatest fears when she first walked in the door being passing on her anxiety condition to her children and not being able to cope as a mother. At that time, although deep down she would have loved a sibling for her baby, she had dreaded having another child even though her husband was keen.

* * * * *

It is easy for individual fears to take complete control of our lives as they did for Melinda, leaving our lives feeling like a hopeless mess. So many tried methods can fail and leave us feeling so broken we think nothing can fix us; I tried what they told me and it hasn't worked, so how sick must I be?

Sometimes we need to keep searching until we find that way to tame fear that works.

The road to taming fear is not always easy. It can be challenging at times, as Melinda would agree.

The key, as Melinda found, was to persist no matter how hard it gets. To face what you don't want to or have avoided for far too long – to finally sit down with our worst fears and befriend them.

The following steps help us resolve our fears – finally tame them – by learning to know and befriend them.

Before we begin, I should point out that the way I help people like Melinda resolve fears in person is somewhat different from how we will do it here. In person, we can ask questions as we go. We can be more flexible in the steps, and tackle previously hidden and more powerful fears that may appear during the sessions as they arise. To compensate for your inability to ask questions, I recommend that you return to previous steps as you require if a new fear arises. For example, if you are at step 5 and your find a more profound fear has arisen, feel free to start steps 1 to 4 again and answer them in your own time.

I have learned from personal experience and by helping others resolve their fears for over a decade that it is easier to rewrite the fear staring us in the face. It is the most powerful. It is easier to rewrite than one in the distance or the one we think is causing the problem. We can think of it as the brain saying this is the most critical fear right now; we need to fix this first. Try to resolve other fears, and we will just have the most potent fear keep showing up and getting in our way. It is better to listen to the brain and go with its priorities, or it becomes more challenging to tame our fears.

As we work to resolve our fears, it is essential to remember the fundamental secret of what the brain wants for the fear to go away: a plan or acceptance. All the following steps are to give the brain what it wants to let the fear go.

How will we know fear is resolved?

You will know. For example, when I've achieved resolution, I often find I take a deep sigh. I feel a bit stupid, wondering why I didn't see that before; it was so obvious. You may have a different experience of the fear leaving you, but you will know it is tamed.

Our approach will be gentle and persistent. We will follow clear steps. There is no rush; take your time. Take each action as you are ready, preferably in order. Try not to miss a step, or you may make it harder for yourself. The steps are in this order for a reason. We will work on one fear at a time.

*****

> **CRITICAL POINT**
>
> We must persist. As with many of our most worthwhile endeavours, we gain the most by sticking with them and not giving up or considering defeat.

I get it: fear makes us terribly uncomfortable. We don't like the feeling. We want it to go away, NOW! That is normal and OK. Fears are supposed to make us feel uncomfortable, horrible or completely overwhelmed, but be reassured that the fear will not harm us, no matter how bad it feels. To help make a fear manageable, I like to think of our fear as being like a giant balloon monster.

Suppose we come across a giant, scary monster. It looks real and about to rip us to shreds. What is our natural reaction, what do our instincts tell us we should do?

Run like Hell!

So, we do. We're off! See ya!

How does the giant, scary monster respond?

You guessed it. It chases us.

So, we run, and we run, and we run, hoping it will fall behind or, better still, disappear. For a while, the monster isn't as noticeable.

Then, there it is. Only this time, the monster is often bigger and scarier than we remember; it's grown.

So, what do we do?

Yep, we're off! Bye now.

This can go on for quite a while until, finally, we are so exhausted that we don't have a choice; we have to face it. Unfortunately, we can't keep running and hiding; the fear monster always seems to find us.

But our fear monster isn't a real, big and scary monster. It is, instead, a balloon monster. It is a monster that looks real on the outside, but get inside it and we find it is full of hot air. It is nothing like it appears on the outside.

It's a bit like when we meet an imposing stranger with tattoos, and we don't like tats; people in tats scare us. But once we get to know the person and can finally see the goodness in their heart, our fears about them go away.

For now, you might just have to take my word for it when I say our fear monster is not as scary as it appears to be. The key is to persist until we see beyond fear's scary mask. You will see what this all means in practice in a moment.

We will use our balloon monster more later.

> ### CRITICAL POINT
> Another point worth noting: we shouldn't be disappointed if we don't get immediate results. We may need to try more than once before we access the fear sufficiently to rewrite it. Also, some fears are deeply ingrained and hide other fears within them that may need resolving first.

I also like to think of fears as a tree of fears. Many fears come from fearful incidents in our past that then grew many branches of fears. Until we get to the primary fearful incident – the main branch – the other fears that divided from the main one will keep coming back.

For example, our first fear of being socially humiliated or bullied may be associated with primary school. We may start out resolving the fear of being shamed or ridiculed at work and, in doing so, trigger and access the more profound fear from the bullying at school. Until we explore and rewrite the fear from school, we can expect other social fears, such as those at work that branched from it, to keep showing up. The initial fear may be so powerful, and we may have suppressed it for so long that accessing it might take time and patience. That is OK.

Once we have learned the steps to resolve our fear, we will apply them as part of a mini-workbook. As mentioned, this will offer a useful summary and practical tips.

CHAPTER 10

FEARS BE GONE!

Melinda was apprehensive and unsure how facing and resolving her fears would go. I could see it in her body language: arms crossed in front of her, legs crisscrossed, leaning forward and seeming quite agitated. It was to be expected. If we seek to resolve a fear, it is normal to have these feelings. After all, what we are about to do is unfamiliar, and we now know how our brain reacts to that. I knew if I spent time reassuring her, she would feel even more scared: how bad must it be if I need reassurance? Better, I found, to be matter of fact and get straight into it.

Learning to tame fears from a book differs from doing it in person with a therapist. Rest assured, our aim is to help you resolve fears safely and in as non-threatening a way as possible. We don't just rush in and try to tackle them head on, otherwise some of us can be so terrified we'll never try to tame them again. Slow and steady is best. Take your time.

If the fears aren't so bad, excellent. It is better to over plan in case they are severe than to be too lax and make us feel worse.

No matter the severity of the fear, a potent strategy to resolving fear is being inquisitive and gradually wanting to know them as you might a new friend. Where did you come from? That's interesting; what made you do that? What bothers you the most? We will learn to converse with our fears in a moment. Ultimately, the fear is our friend; we just haven't learned how to talk with it properly yet so it can stop being such an annoyance.

The process of resolving a fear will be broken into three parts or stages. First, we start with preparation, much like we did for learning mindfulness meditations earlier. Then, once we are settled and well prepared, we will learn to chat with the fear, to resolve it. Finally, in case that hasn't worked, or we get stuck, we will learn some supplemental ways to tame the fear not mentioned in the stages above. It's always good to have some extra tricks up our sleeve just in case.

> **CRITICAL POINT**
>
> A warning before we begin. Please do not bypass or look past the preparation section and go straight to facing and rewriting your fear, such as heading straight for the mini-workbook. We wouldn't jump out of a plane with a parachute without a pre-jump check and preparation first, would we? Not unless we want to be splattered on the ground. The following preparation is there for your benefit; please take it seriously.

Remember, we aren't about to walk on the moon without a spacesuit. So, we can take a deep breath. This is much safer than some risky venture. Besides, having seen the worst that fear can dish at us, I'm confident we can make progress together.

Stage 1: Preparations

Step 1. Find a Safe Place

It is next to impossible to resolve a fear if our fear bomb has gone off, if we are triggered and scared out of our wits. The key to resolving fears is facing them on our terms, not theirs. The time to deal with a fear of heights, for instance, isn't when we've just been thrown over the side of a tall building dangling by a flimsy rope; though some might disagree. I prefer a gentler approach to timing.

To help us tackle a fear, we first need to feel safe and know we can stop the fear distressing us if it gets too much. We need physical safety, and we need a way to dial down the fear volume to reduce the anxiety anytime we need to.

Our task is to find/create two kinds of safe places: a physically safe place and a mentally safe place or retreat.

A Physically Safe Place

Find a place where you feel safe and secure and won't be disturbed, as we did in our preparation for meditation (see Chapter 4). Being disturbed even for a short time slows down progress and can be very annoying.

A Mentally Safe Place

Imagine the safest place you can. It can be from your past, such as sitting under a tree was for me. Perhaps you have read of a place that sounds calm, tranquil and ideal. Your mentally safe place is your retreat, and no one needs to know about it. They key is that you know it brings up a sense of safety and peace for you.

Now, close your eyes and visualise yourself in this place of complete safety. Notice as much detail as you can and observe how it feels. Embrace the greens of the grass and the blues of the water and sky. Feel the grittiness of the sand between your toes. Smell the alluring freshness of the spring breeze. The more granularity you give your mentally safe place the more substantial and powerful it will be. Rest there for a few minutes, so you are familiar with it. Give it a name:

My mentally safe place is …………………………………..

If our fear gets too much, we know at any time we can go to our mentally safe place. It can be a good way of temporarily calming the anxiety until we have resolved it. Try not to use it unless you need to. Going that bit further and allowing us to be uncomfortable with fear can be a powerful way to resolve it. Remember, you control whether you go to this mentally safe place. You will get to know when to use it best.

> **Make it a rule: if your fear is not resolved by the end of your attempt, then finish your session in your mentally safe place. Then, stay there for a while, like a meditation, before you return to everyday life.**

Resting in our mentally safe place is a mental technique that is especially useful when facing and dealing with significant fears or traumas of our past. Many trauma therapists teach their clients to find this mentally safe place before rewriting the fear.

Practise being in your mentally safe place. It can help you even when you aren't trying to put your fears in the outbox. It can bring peace to an otherwise hectic day.

Step 2. Name It to Tame It

In the beginning, Melinda had a veritable fear-scape of fears that were terrorising her. When I initially asked her what she was afraid of, chief among her fears was the thought, as mentioned earlier, of never getting better. It was having to be like this for the rest of her life or, worse, feeling she can't go on and leaving her daughter motherless and her husband a widow – that she'd have to end her life. The thought of fear always controlling you or driving you to an early grave is a common fear I find among those suffering severe anxiety. It is widespread among those who have tried other treatments that didn't work, those who say they don't know how much longer they can keep doing this. I knew we needed to find and tame the underlying fear that started this all off for Melinda. Melinda wasn't always like this; the anxiety and panic had been present for under two years.

Naming a fear isn't always easy. It isn't uncommon for anxiety sufferers to not know what they are afraid of. In fact, some claim to have had anxiety or a high level of fear their whole life and can't name any particular fear or fears that bother them. How this happens and how to tame fear in that case we will discuss in Chapter 12. Sometimes, the fear controlling us isn't what it appears to be; it can be more profound, as with the earlier example of how a fear of humiliation at work began in childhood, not from work itself.

What triggered Melinda's fear? It was a social fear that first started during a family function with her husband's parents. Melinda remembered it clearly. She wasn't feeling well during the meal and didn't know why; there was no reason to feel this way. Soon she felt flushed, her heart was racing and, very embarrassed, she felt she had to leave the table. The mild discomfort passed, but then it returned at work – the same sensations all over again.

Having health industry training, Melinda wondered if something was seriously medically wrong with her. She was imagining the worst. The downside of working in the health industry is we can either worry we have something terrible or think a significant problem is trivial. On the other hand, the benefit of working in health is that you know the best people to seek professional advice from.

To Melinda's frustration, no one could find a reason for her symptoms. But she was sure they were missing something serious. She was sure whatever illness they couldn't find would leave her daughter motherless. The mere thought of such a scenario terrified her again, and her heart started racing as before. No matter what she told herself, no matter how much self-reassurance, the fear would not leave. She was suffering terribly.

The fear that most controlled her, the root fear feeding all the others, wasn't that she was afraid her anxiety would be her undoing. Instead, it was the terror that a physical illness would, and she could do nothing about it.

To name our fear means finding the fear at the heart of our anxieties, recognising it and putting a name to it. Then, to describe what it is precisely we are afraid of. If it is evident, great; we have a fear we can work with. If it isn't, it may take some time to show itself as we work on whatever fear we have in front of us.

OK, I know my fear. It is on my list.

You have named your fear and are satisfied it is the one most bothering you. So, we will go with that.

What if I'm not sure what my ultimate fear is. Yes, I listed it, but I'm having doubts. Or I'm not sure what my fear is now, but I know I still have one?

Here are some rules to help you name your fear.

Rules to Make Naming a Fear Easier and Honest

Never Let Anyone Tell You What Your Fear Is

Fear is your personal experience. Only you know whether you are truly afraid of something. You know by how you feel. If specific thoughts, places or people trigger a fear response, they represent a fear. If they don't trigger a feeling of fear, then they are not a fear for you, no matter what anyone says. Trust in your feelings.

One problem our brain has when dealing with fear is it can be coached into believing a trauma and associated fear happened when it didn't. So don't let others coach you into believing something you know not to be true in your heart.

Avoid Denying a Fear

Denying your fear out of ego or pride doesn't make it disappear. 'A person like me isn't afraid of spiders. Don't be ridiculous.' By denying our fears, we suppress them, making them harder to find, recognise and rewrite. Denying fears also ensures the fears keep influencing us, making them stronger than they need to be. Denying we have a fear doesn't work.

Try not to deny your fears. Be open to the many fears that might be there.

And try not to judge your fears: 'Oh, this is a terrible fear. I shouldn't feel that way.' Fears are neither good nor evil. If we judge our worries, we are more likely to deny them.

Fears are just a response. Try to search with curiosity what triggered the response: what brought it on, what events happened and what scenarios we have started to worry about that we didn't before. For Melinda the trigger was feeling unwell at the dinner. The scenario that scared her was that she had a severe illness that would kill her, leaving her child motherless.

Don't get upset or angry with yourself for responding as you did. Remember, our brain is simply responding as it was made to do.

*****

To help remind you what fear you are dealing with, write down the fear that most bothers you here:

The fear that most bothers me is

....

If you need to change it later, that is OK.

Step 3. Reality-check the Fairies and Unicorns

Don't forget that our brain is an excellent fantasy-making machine. Every fear we come up with and every scenario it creates is ultimately a fantasy. Our brains make many stories, some more realistic and valuable than others. Some are ridiculous, but we can still fall for them, accept them as legitimate or genuine.

The problem is, as we noted earlier, when it comes to making us afraid, our brain doesn't know what is real until it happens. It doesn't know the difference between real possibilities and complete fantasy. So, our brain can potentially make us afraid of the equivalent of nasty fairies and angry, pink unicorns. We don't need to let it.

A quick way to lower the number of our fears is, for each, to simply and honestly ask: Is this fear realistic? Is it?

I can imagine the moon exploding and landing on my home or medical practice in the next hour. Does that mean I should get in my car and take off inland or up the coast? That would be silly.

Just because our mind can develop a fear doesn't mean we have to act on it. It doesn't mean it is worth our effort to develop a plan. If we can acknowledge in our hearts that the imagined fear is pure fantasy and absurd, we can accept it for what it is: a waste of our time and energy. Once we accept this, the fear will pass.

Are you being terrorised by nasty fairies and pink unicorns? Is the moon about to land on your house?

The same skill also works well with new fears as they show up. Ask if they are realistic the moment they show up. The key, though, is not to try to rationalise it away and just say it is silly, as that won't work. The way to make the brain let the fear go is to engage with it emotionally, play out the simulation it has created, and question its realism and worth. Is it really worth considering? Really? Simply using logic to dismiss the fear as silly doesn't engage the brain's emotional stimulation and, hence, doesn't make the fear disappear. We will use the brain's emotionally engaged simulator to resolve anxiety more soon.

Roberto, an apprentice plumber in his early twenties, found this strategy especially helpful. We had discussed the secrets of fears we mentioned earlier. I didn't see him for months and then he unexpectedly came in for an unrelated medical condition. I asked him about his anxiety, and he dismissed it; it's not a problem. Instead, he found that asking two questions helped him settle almost all his fears. The first question: is this fear realistic – is it likely to happen? The second question: will it really matter in ten years? Just two questions, and he'd mastered his anxiety. He was delighted.

His use of the second question is a strategy we will discuss more in a moment.

Go back through your list of fears you wrote at the beginning. Are any of them totally unrealistic? Be honest. Run the emotional simulation and see. Imagine and feel them. If they are unrealistic, ask, honestly, are they really worth my time?

How do you feel about the list of fears now? Do you still have one or more fears we need to resolve?

If you do, then let us move on. But, if you don't, you may still find the other fear-taming skills we are about to learn to be helpful if you need other options to tame fear when your usual strategies don't work.

Like Roberto, I have had many people tell me they find it very useful to simply ask whether their fear is realistic. Checking whether fear is realistic may sound like a simple technique, but it can be a potent fear-taming tool. It can resolve many fears very quickly.

Why does this skill work?

Remembering the secrets of fear we mentioned earlier, this approach offers our brain both acceptance and a plan: the fundamentals of what it wants in order to resolve any fear.

For example, by checking to see if our fear is realistic, we are engaging our brain's emotional simulator. We are playing it out in our mind. This lets our brain create possible plans: what might happen and what we might do. This shows the brain that the plans are useless; we can do nothing. It is a baseless fear and too unlikely to ever happen. Our brain accepts the fear isn't worth our energy.

Essentially, we are talking to our brain and showing it what we want it to see with images that have added feelings attached. We talk using our brain's emotional simulator. We are talking to our brain in a familiar language to see what type of scenarios it is prepared to accept.

Try it. Whenever a new fear comes along, ask yourself 'Is this really likely to happen? Is it really worth my time and attention?' Explore using your emotional simulator. Be honest. What do you feel?

OK, we've checked whether our fear is real. Now what?

We work on the following steps to tame it.

CHAPTER 11

FROM FEAR TO FRIEND

Stage 2: Hi! Time For a Chat!

For Melinda, recognising and sitting with her fear was horrible; she tried to avoid it at all costs. Then, as she began to feel more anxiety, she wanted to sit with it even less. This is where learning to visualise the fear as a giant balloon monster helped. It allowed her to take a step back from the fear and see it differently – to rewrite it.

It is well known that when fear kicks in, a part of the brain called the amygdala becomes active and sends signals to the front of the brain – the prefrontal cortex that does the planning – and shuts it down. That means when we are severely afraid, we struggle to solve complex problems or to make sense of what is going on. This is the brain saying act, don't think. We must do something NOW, not analyse how many teeth are in the shark's mouth or what species it is. We need to get out of the water.

Seeing our fear as a giant balloon monster can help our brain detach from the fear enough to allow us to keep thinking while feeling the fear. The brain can do it just enough to allow us to change the fear on the inside, to reconsider and rewrite the scenario that is making us so afraid.

It's like being so nervous in an exam that our minds go blank. Once we settle down, we more effortlessly remember what we have learnt, allowing us to solve the problems on paper or on the computer in front of us. Stay too afraid, and our mind remains blank.

We now have the name of your fear monster; you wrote it down. Now we will work on simple steps to get to know that monster and find the friend within it who is trying to warn, prepare and keep us safe. We will let it know we have listened and are thankful for its help.

The first step in getting to know our fear is to stop running. It's hard to chat with someone while running away from them.

Step 4. Have a Sit-down

I would like you to sit down and say hello to your fear. Yes, really.

Imagine two chairs facing each other in a big room. We sit in one. Then, taking a deep breath, we make space for the fear and ask it to sit in the chair opposite us a few metres away.

Yes, we feel uncomfortable with it so close. That is normal. Just sit and rest with it a moment. Let it be there. Let each of you get used to being in each other's company without heading for the hills.

Say, hello, fear, how are you going? Don't expect much of an answer yet; the fear is still getting used to you giving it attention without having to run after you.

By sitting with our fear, we begin to face it, and we finally give ourselves a chance to listen to it and help give it what it needs for it to go away.

The bottom line is we cannot tame a fear until we face it. Yes, it can be difficult at first. I don't like facing my fears initially either, and I've faced countless, some extreme. Just take your time. Don't get distracted or leave the fear. Hold your fear in your presence. Be inquisitive. Want to get to know it.

If you find sitting with it too difficult, an alternative is to write about it. Write a short story as if you were someone else facing and sitting with this same fear. Describe what the fear is like and how it affects your character. Let it know the troubles it has caused and continues to. Let it know it is time to respectfully listen to each other and finally be friends, to help us see we are on the same side. Later we will explore how we can use this technique and other similar methods to unlock and confront our terror.

Step 5. Have the Chat and Ask the Primary Question

Now that we are sitting, we can have a chat. We can begin the chat by getting to the point by asking: What do you want from me for you to go away?

Ask the question honestly and listen for an answer. Be open to what it has to share.

Surprisingly, our fear may answer us straight away, often with an image or visualisation of what it wants us to do.

> **It is crucial to note that fear doesn't communicate in words. Instead, it uses images and feelings.**

We shouldn't be shocked if we get a reply. Commonly, our fear will quickly remind us of what we already know but don't want to deal with or face because it seems too difficult or inconvenient. It isn't easy, and we like easy.

Remember, all our fear is asking for is a plan or acceptance: what are you going to do about it, or do we accept there really is nothing we can do at all? It wants to know that, in the end, we will be OK.

For instance, if the fear concerns finances, maybe downsizing is the only way to stop feeling stressed about money. On the other hand, if we are afraid of a bully, perhaps we just need to face the bully. We'll explore these two examples in more detail in a moment.

Anne, a loving parent of a nine-year-old daughter, learned this approach. It was her favourite.

At the beginning of every day, Anne would ask her mind, what am I afraid of, and what does my fear need for it to go away? Then she would open her mind to the answer.

She told me that, intuitively, she already knew what the answer would be, but in the past had dismissed or ignored it. Not anymore. Now she would take seriously the solutions she'd been shown and take practical, concrete steps to enact them.

For instance, if Anne felt afraid before a job interview, she'd make sure she was better prepared. If she was fearful of her ability to pay the bills, she'd look to find a better-paying job or for more work. Anne wouldn't let the fear fester; she'd be on it right away with things to do. Sometimes the solutions weren't obvious and would take a day or so to show up, but she always asked the question every morning, without fail.

Anne also said she focused on the solution rather than dwelling on the problem: the fear. She said this approach immediately began to reduce and resolve many of her fears. It worked well for her.

Do you have a solution to your fear?

If you do, write down at least four practical steps you can take to enact them.

Four practical steps to resolve my fear.

1. ....
2. ....
3. ....
4. ....

What if we can't find a plan, a solution or a way to see the situation that lets us know we will be OK?

We can do one of two things: we can work on other ways to find that plan (such as those we will learn by calling fear's bluff in a moment) or see if acceptance works.

Will Acceptance Work?

Like Ellie trying to keep her children safe, can you accept that there is nothing you can do that will realistically make a difference to what you are afraid of? Does acceptance tame your fear balloon monster, make it flutter deflated into the distance?

Remember, we can't fake acceptance. If the brain thinks there is the slightest thing it can do to change the outcome, it will keep making you afraid until you give it the plan it thinks must exist.

I can't find acceptance. I just can't.

That's fine. It is OK if we can't find that acceptance; not all fears allow it.

Keep asking the fear – as if it was that balloon monster in front of you – the question: what do you want from me to go away? Give it time. It might be getting over the shock of you actually talking to it. Perhaps you, like Anne, should ask those questions of your fears every morning. Then, after a while it will get used to showing you more readily, as it did for Anne.

What if I make no progress and the fear doesn't let me know what will fix it?

Then we work with it to create the plan or acceptance in other ways, such as calling its bluff.

Step 6. Call Fear's Bluff

If only facing fear was enough for it to dissolve into the distance forever. Unfortunately, it's not.

Just stepping in front of the balloon monster won't resolve it. But letting it flow through us like a ghost or stepping inside it and looking around when we are inside it almost certainly will.

If you have a fear that you struggle to resolve, I can guarantee you have not let your fear give it its best shot. And you definitely haven't explored inside it in all its detail. Instead, you may have avoided it, walked or ran to get further away from it, hung around it or skirted the edges. You have not tackled it on your terms.

Just to be clear, getting angry with a fear of doing something despite being afraid (such as parachuting if you are scared of heights) isn't the same as stepping inside it. And Batman fans, we can't resolve a fear by adopting its symbol, as Batman did in response to his fear of bats. From what I know of the Bruce Wayne character, he certainly hasn't learned to step inside his fear. All those billions, and he still hasn't seen a therapist.

Mind you, no one can blame us for not stepping inside a fear, since even just approaching a fear on the outside is bad enough; it gets worse the closer we get. But it is this next step that makes all the difference.

One of the fastest ways to resolve a fear is to call its bluff.

What does it mean to call a fear's bluff? And why does it make fears go away and stay away?

Calling fear's bluff means imagining that the worst-case fear scenario had come true and letting ourselves feel the fear in all its raw fury, not holding back. Then we either let the fear flow through us or we explore it while experiencing it. We look from within at what our options are that could resolve our concerns and see the fear in ways we never have before.

There are two main ways to call our fear's bluff: a direct approach and an indirect approach. The direct approach can be the most challenging, but it can also be the fastest and tame the worst fears imaginable. The indirect approach takes longer, but can offer enormous insight into who we are both as individuals and as human beings.

What is the direct approach?

Direct Approach

You may recall at the beginning I described how, during my internal journey in my twenties, I let the worst possible fears imaginable have their way with me. I let them give me their worst – all the demons, hellfire, you name it; I didn't let them hold back. Then, surprisingly, I found the fear dissolved. Soon after, I could see fear differently, and it no longer controlled me. This was the direct approach.

I remember a lady who suffered from terrible fears from past traumas, having failed all therapies over many years, saying to herself one day, I'm over this shit. F*** it. I'm not going to let these fears control me anymore. She'd been holding back from dealing with her fears head on, and it hadn't worked. So, she allowed them to go ballistic. For a while, she felt very uncomfortable. Then, peace.

Think of the direct way of calling fear's bluff as your balloon monster being a ghost. Let it walk inside you and give you every bit of fear, anger and frustration it has. Let it have no limits. Just sit there as it does its thing. Soon its energy fades; it can't keep it up. By the end, it floats out the other side, having taken all your feelings of fear towards it with it; the fear/s are tamed.

Maybe it's time to get fed up with your fear. Instead of stopping it from making you feel horrible, let it do the opposite. Let it be free, and see how long it lasts.

The mistake we can make here is holding back, even a little. Then it is like our ghost balloon monster has left something behind, and our fear remains.

If you are not prepared to commit to this approach, do not give it a try since it can discourage you; oh, great, another strategy that didn't work. We must be prepared to fully experience and hold our fear for it to work. If you prefer, you can do this in the safety of a consult with your therapist.

Is this approach for everyone?

No. For starters, not everyone is fed up enough with their fear to be motivated to try.

If this approach isn't for you, that is alright. There is a less direct approach.

Indirect Approach

We can use an indirect approach to achieve a similar result to directly calling our fear's bluff: with curiosity.

Here we imagine our giant balloon monster – fear – and instead of standing in front of it and being terrified by it, we step inside it and look around. In effect, we imagine the worst case our brain has come up with comes true, and ask ourselves what we will do. Instead of avoiding fear or skirting around the edges, we face it honestly and know it intimately.

How does this approach work?

By stepping inside the monster, we are accessing the simulation scenario that triggers our fear. Then, we are rewriting the scenario by being curious and exploring it from different angles from the inside – adding more information and perspectives. Finally, we choose to see the fear more completely and realistically.

A helpful way to step inside fear and explore it so our brain sees the different perspectives is by imagining the worst case. Then we allow ourselves to feel the fear it brings and begin asking questions.

Consider the following three examples.

You Are Terrified You Can't Pay the Bills and Will Lose Your Home
To call this fears' bluff, we imagine losing the home: our worst fear. We let ourselves feel the experience, and as we do, we ask questions about the fear and the scenario. Some helpful questions can include:

- Yes, it feels terrible, but will I be OK and still living alright in five – or ten – years?
- Will my family and other essential people in my life still be there and care for me?
- Are the family most valuable or the home and the mortgage?
- I know how to succeed. I have in the past. Don't you think I can do it again if I need to?
- Can I rebuild, perhaps start anew? We might end up with a better home.

- If, in the worst-case scenario, the most important people still love and support me, how is that such a terrible worst case?

Many of us are terrified of having to downsize. We may worry our family thinks less of us for having to go with less, though we probably haven't even talked with them to find out. So instead, we make any number of assumptions in the fantasy of our worst case. Still, we don't challenge any of the premises and explore them. They make us too uncomfortable.

Calling our fear's bluff means we don't just fixate on the fear. Instead, we explore and challenge it from the inside by examining different assumptions and perspectives. The more alternatives we see, the more we offer our brain a realistic picture to create the plan or acceptance it wants.

You are Petrified Your Partner Will Leave You
Calling this fear's bluff is imaging our partner does leave. Then we look to questions that help us see beyond it, such as:

- Could I do anything more than what I am doing in the relationship? If there is more that I could do, then what is it?
- Are we really that compatible? Honestly.
- Why am I staying? Does my partner meet my needs?
- Am I just staying because I'm afraid to be alone?
- Am I dependent on them? Could I make it on my own – even thrive – if I needed to?
- Do I need to see a lawyer and/or therapist to help clarify my options? Am I just afraid of the unknown?
- If we share all our friends, could I make new friends?

- If I looked back in ten years, how would I see our breakup, if it were to happen? Would I see it as an opportunity, a life turning point, a blessing, a learning experience or perhaps a challenge that made me stronger?
- Would breaking up and learning from the mistakes of this relationship set me up for an even better relationship in the future?

When we are afraid of breakups, we can naturally fear losing what we cherish or even fear the unknown; what will it be like without them? In this circumstance, our brain wants to know what we can do, whether we will eventually be OK, and whether there is anything we need to prepare for. If the brain is scared, it is almost certainly focusing on the negatives, not the potential positives.

But I don't see any positives.

Then we aren't being realistic, are we? Of course, there are always possible positives from even the worst experiences. Still, we won't see them unless we let ourselves be open to – or search for – them. Seeing the good, the bad and the indifferent possibilities offers us a more realistic way of seeing the scenario we are afraid of, rather than just the negatives we have been focused on.

Of course, no longer being terrified our partner will leave us liberates us and our relationship. It means we can be ourselves and not have to be a slave to their whims or moods. It means we don't have to spend our time trying to please them. It means we can spend time together confident we are there because we both want to be. Who wants to be in a relationship where they can't be themselves? How stifling and unsatisfying would that be?

You are Afraid of Bullying at Work or School

Calling this fear's bluff means we imagine we are bullied. Now what? With this fear, we have several approaches. We can ask:

- What can we do to fix this?
- Is this my fault? Do I need to change or is this more about the other person? The other person may be a sociopath, for example, and would target us anyway, no matter what we did. Or maybe they are being bullied or were as a child. After all, if we are bullied, we are more likely to do it to others.
- Is this position worth it? What are my options? List and research your job/career choices. Then, develop a longer-term plan. A job change may be in order.
- Do I need to confront the bully? What are the outcomes I can prepare for? Who can I call upon for support?
- What am I worried about most when facing the bully? What is my worst case?
- Will I lose my friends and family if I finally confront this person and maybe lose my job because of it?
- Am I most afraid of losing my job over this or how others might see me? Would my real friends think less of me if I lose or change jobs?
- Does this fear of confronting bullies go back a long way? Do I struggle to stand up for myself?
- Am I confident I can find another job if I need to? Have I looked?

Bullying seems to be common; I regularly see people suffering from it. Bullying can trigger many fear scenarios, such as fear of being hurt, humiliated or ostracised, of losing our job or of it impacting our career or family life. Many fears related to bullying often go back to the first time it happened, leaving deep emotional scars and the anxieties that go with them. Unfortunately, the first time we are bullied could be in childhood; childhood bullying is too common.

The point is, even in fear of being bullied, our brain is still just after a plan or acceptance. Can I accept that I will be bullied and not make that change or stop or will I take action to do something about it? Even if there is the slightest idea that you can do something, the fear will keep bugging you until you have finalised a plan – what you will actually do about it.

By asking the bullying monster lots of questions, we help our brains see what these alternative actions might be and what the outcomes might look like.

What if we still have a fear of bullying from childhood? How do we change that?

I, too, suffered lots of childhood bullying, and to my shame now, I did some myself. The question that helped me better resolve my emotional pains and fears was if the other children came from families that taught kindness, compassion and tolerance would I have been bullied? The answer was no.

Answering this question helped me to more realistically see the forces at play that led to me being treated so poorly. It helped me realise that children reflect their parents; we have very little insight and awareness when we are young. By realising this, I could see the bullying wasn't my fault. This was important to know.

Why is it so important to know the bullying wasn't my fault?

It allows us to better see our role in the bullying without negative judgement, without being hard on ourselves. It also makes the whole scenario of the bullying more predictable.

Was there really anything I could have done as a child to stop the bullying?

Probably not, since we can only do what we've been taught. If we are different, are treated poorly at home or have never learned how to be friends, of course being bullied is more likely.

Can I change characteristics within me to avoid bullying in the future, such as learning how to be better friends?

Sure, you can. (See the 10 needs of friendship mentioned in Chapter 7.)

By asking my fear just one question, I gave my brain more information to create a more realistic scenario. Hence, it then has a plan of what it can and can't do in a similar scenario next time. I have let it create both a plan and acceptance. Once I did this, the fear balloon monster of bullying from childhood fluttered away, and I felt at peace with that part of my past.

How much of your fear of bullying is about you and your behaviours and fears? How much is about the perpetrator? How have they been treated in the past, and what are their fears and insecurities? Is it primarily about you or about them? Now, what are you going to do about it?

*****

Melinda calling her fear's bluff was next to impossible, but she did it. We imagined her with a severe and terminal illness. But, we asked, is there anything she could do to prevent this? Probably not; we can only live healthy lives as best we can. Would it be terribly sad to leave your daughter behind? Absolutely. But we might be hit by a car tomorrow; none of us know when our time is up. Wouldn't it be better, then, to make the most of what we have now and hold them as most precious, no matter our health? Melinda agreed, making the most of the moments to cherish now would feel better than spending them worrying about things she could do nothing about. We explored each scenario, imagining it in detail.

In our short chat, helping her face and converse with her fear, Melinda learned to see her fear more realistically and from different points of view. In the process, she developed plans of what she might do and acceptance for what was beyond her control. Her fear then began to fade away.

Ideally, we should call a fear's bluff early, before it becomes too big and scary. That means, as soon as we notice our fear, we name it, sit down with it and ask it questions, rather than let it fester for months or years as Melinda did.

What if I call my fear's bluff, and it still hasn't gone? What if I don't feel any relief?

Don't be disappointed if you don't find a resolution of fear in one sitting. Instead, come back to it and work on it again at another time, perhaps days or a week later. In the meantime, your brain will be going over what you have shown it. Then, it will start to look for a solution on its own. You may even have a moment of inspiration when you find suddenly, without planning it, you see the answer, and the weight of the fear lifts, like one of those aha moments.

Suppose I am still not getting anywhere, and it has been weeks. What do I do?

We go back through steps two to six.

We name the fear. We ask what is it I am actually afraid of?

As we've noted, many fears have other parts. Perhaps there are other fears in this one we need to work on first. For example, Melinda had fears within fears. She was afraid of illness and terrified of her anxiety, which was her response to her fear of the disease and what it would mean for her family. We could have called the bluff of the fear of being afraid of her anxiety and might have made some headway. Still, then the fear of being ill and of leaving her daughter without a mother would have come up and needed to be dealt with too. The deeper fears would have just kept creating strong fear reactions and made her even more convinced her anxiety would never leave her.

If calling the bluff of the fear you are resolving isn't working, ask if there are any other fears attached to it, other fears that it has been built upon. Then search with your feelings to see what those fears might be.

Like we mentioned earlier, fears are often like a tree. The fears grow from the big branches, and smaller ones grow from them. If we don't tackle the fear of the main branches, the other fears will remain, and we struggle to tame the fears in front of us.

Keep calling the fear's bluff. Get to know it intimately, like sitting down and getting to know the intimacies of a close friend. We don't judge. Instead, we get curious and see how the pieces fit together, how A led to B, led to C, and so on.

The more we look inside our fears, the more we find to allow us to understand them. The more we understand them, the more familiar the fears become and the more able we are to tame them.

What if I don't want to, or I'm not ready to call my fear's bluff? Are there other ways to help the brain resolve the fear with a plan or acceptance?

Yes.

The next three steps offer us other powerful skills. If the above steps are the preliminary and main techniques, the next three can be considered supplementary.

CHAPTER 12

MAGIC AND MIND TRICKS

Stage 3: Supplementary Skills

Once most of Melinda's fears had been tamed, she also realised she'd lost her confidence at work. This was to be expected since her work became associated with possibly having a panic episode at any moment. However, most of the fear wasn't while she was working. Once she was busy there was almost no anxiety and she was fine, but before work she found her fear levels rising. We called this fear's bluff too, working through worst cases, but it didn't seem to help much. Then we successfully tamed the fear using some simulator magic.

Step 7. Rehearse Success: Simulator Magic

Fear of failing is common. Just like Melinda, we all feel it or have felt it at some time. Perhaps we've been afraid of failing at a sporting event, doing poorly in a speech or screwing up in a meeting or exam. Being afraid to fail is normal. But when we were fearful of getting it wrong, what were we rehearsing in our mind: our failure or our success? In other words, when we were worried about failing, were we imagining how it would go well or poorly?

To worry about failing is to rehearse our failure.

What does rehearsing failure mean, and how do I stop it?

You will recall our brain's job is to rehearse the future. It does this by laying down nerve connections and pathways that will determine what we will do – future memories. In effect, our brain uses an inbuilt simulator. It prepares us for what will happen by simulating it before it happens. So, for example, simply imagining failure can make failure more likely to happen.

How can I simply imagine my failure making failure my reality?

If we spend hours and hours imagining how we will fail, we are laying down connections in our brain telling it how to react in that time and place. We are rehearsing how we will miss the shot, freeze up in front of others during the speech or get so flustered during the exam that we cannot think. We are teaching our brain how to react. Our brain is then obliging and doing what we trained it to do in that situation.

Imagine you were an airline pilot. You were taught how to do the wrong things during your emergency simulations, so the plane crashed. You rehearsed this crashing over and over until it became second nature. How do you then expect to react when the emergency happens? In the heat of the moment, your brain will go back to what it knows: the plans it has rehearsed. In an emergency, you will, almost automatically, crash the plane. And it may be very hard for you not to since you haven't planned the alternative; it isn't your more natural rehearsed response.

By Melinda imagining failing at work, she unwittingly rehearsed it, thus increasing the possibility of making mistakes.

So, the cure to a fear of failure is to imagine not failing?

No, that won't work either.

Have you ever told a young child don't jump on the bed? Instead, you leave them alone, and what do they do? Jump on the bed! But I told them!

But what image did we give their brain when we told them not to jump on the bed? The only one you shared was jumping on the bed, so that is what they rehearsed, and that is what they did.

As many parents already know, a better approach to stop the child from jumping on the bed would be to put the image in their mind of doing something we are happy for them to do, like play with the toy cars on the bedroom floor. The toy cars look especially fun right now. I wonder which is fastest if we race them? So now the child has an image of having fun racing the cars, and the notion of jumping on the bed isn't even being considered.

This is why telling someone to not be afraid is equally useless. By telling someone not to be scared, we trigger memories of being afraid. We make the fear stronger or more prominent. We instil in them rehearsing being afraid.

How do I stop my brain rehearsing failure and triggering the fears that go with it?

A significant way of resolving our fear of failure is simple: rehearse our success! To clarify, rehearsing success does not mean vague, irrational, wishful thinking and unrealistic dreaming. In our mind we might rehearse flying like Superman, but no simulations will ever make it real. Instead, by rehearsing success we offer a form of practice of what is within our physical abilities – getting the most from what we've got.

The simulation we run in our brain also satisfies our fear's need for a plan. By rehearsing success, we resolve our fear by giving the brain the plans to succeed.

We prepare for our success using visualisations, perhaps imagining in detail what we will do in our job interview or practising our speech in front of a mirror. These visualisations allow our brain to accept there is nothing more we can reasonably do; we know we are giving it our best.

Once the brain has the plan and acceptance, the fear goes away or will significantly reduce. We may even notice some confidence.

How do I apply rehearsing success as a skill day to day?

Consider the following suggestions you can use when you are nervous before an event, for instance:

- First, recognise that the fear you feel means you are rehearsing your failure. Recognise your anxiety and what scenario you are afraid of.
- Now, imagine the same scenario but only your success, no matter the obstacles.
- Reinforce your success through practice and more practice. If you can, physically do it. Otherwise, simply rehearse the scenario in your mind.

Why is practice critical?

Practice is critical because every time we practise something, we further stabilise the brain connections we use for practising that thing. This makes it more likely those brain connections will be used in the time and place we are preparing for.

But, surely, rehearsing in my mind isn't enough?

A small study compared music students who practised in front of a piano versus those who practised in their mind. Each group practised for the same hours. Then, after a significant time, they checked to see who was better – or worse – at playing the piano, those who physically practised versus those who rehearse in their minds. Which group do you think improved the most? There was no significant difference. It was as though it didn't matter whether we rehearse with a real piano or an imagined one, so long as we spend the time rehearsing.

Rehearsing in our brain creates real changes in the brain. So, when you practise in your mind how you will do well, you are more likely to do well.

What if I rehearse doing well but still feel afraid that I'll fail? What do I do then?

We look at the bigger picture.

Imagine you are a top tennis player, but nothing more; your life, your sense of self is all about you as a tennis player. If you lose at tennis, you aren't just losing a game. It is you losing – and being a loser – as a person; being a loser then defines you.

Now imagine that tennis is only a tiny part of your bigger life. For instance, you are a loving partner of a caring person, you are a great friend to many and a valued member of a community and society. Now, if you lose a game of tennis, you aren't a loser. It was just one game; the game doesn't define you.

If we fear losing everything, that will be a massive fear. If we fear losing just one small part of our life and otherwise our satisfying life can still go on, then we aren't going to be as afraid.

We are all allowed to get a little nervous about failing. It can keep us sharp. The aim is not to lose perspective to the point that the fear of failure becomes so powerful it dominates our life.

* * * * *

Melinda would rehearse every night before work how it would go well on the job the next day, and in the morning she would again imagine that success. If there was an emergency, she had rehearsed what she would do and how well she would do it. If she had some fear, she rehearsed how to settle it. There were no fear episodes at work. The more she succeeded at work, the more she began to realise there was nothing at work to be afraid of. Fear of failure was replaced by confidence in success.

*****

What about fears that make no sense, irrational fears, such as severe fears of spiders, or places that seem safe but make us feel scared for no reason? How do we tame them? One way is to use memory shenanigans.

Step 8. Combat Memory Shenanigans

Imagine you are six years old and tagging along with your mum as she goes to the local department store. It is your first time in the big, strange-smelling building and seeing so much stuff. People are hard to find; the place is mostly empty. Your mum squeezes your hand tightly. She appears agitated and unsettled. Her fear is contagious, and now you feel scared too. Your mother is nervous every time she takes you to this one department store. You have no idea why. Even if your mother isn't with you, you start to feel scared in this one store. But nothing terrible happened. Why should we be frightened of a place where there is no rational reason to be?

Suppose you are terrified of spiders. It's called arachnophobia, the irrational fear of tiny – sometimes not so tiny – eight-legged critters.

To even think of a spider sends shivers down your spine. The last time you saw a real spider, it freaked you out and sent you running from the room. But a spider never hurt me. So why should I be afraid of a spider? I have no bad memories of them?

The answer to why we are afraid in these scenarios is because the fear was laid down as a memory. We remember that this is what made us afraid last time.

Consider the two examples.

In the department store, we learned our fear from our mother. Fear is contagious. When one of us is afraid, the rest of us often are too; we noted this earlier. It is a good survival strategy that if our parents are scared, we learn what they are afraid of and become fearful of it. After all, they know more about surviving this world than we do. We are young and yet to learn what can kill us. Our mother taught our brain a fear link, an association between the department store and fear. It is like attaching sticky chewing gum to a tennis ball. Every time we pick up the ball, there is the gum.

Of course, nature assumes our parent has a good reason to be afraid. What if they never learned to tame fears. What if this is a fear from a bad experience never resolved, such as being badly humiliated or being held up? What if they learned this fear from their parents and now are also making us afraid for no reason? It is an irrational fear.

Similarly, the fear of spiders can be taught by our parents. They may have gone ballistic when they saw a spider near us as a younger child and terrified us. They may be terrified of spiders themselves.

It doesn't matter how our parents pass on their fear of something; once we learn the fear from our parents, it stays there until we die or we resolve it.

Many fears that don't make sense to us and don't readily settle when we call their bluff can be fears that have been learned but have no rational reason to still be there. The problem is our brain doesn't know not to be afraid. It just knows walk into that department store, panic; see a spider, freak out!

* * * * *

I put phobias, such as fear of spiders, into the category of fear memories. This is because to fix them, we use a common approach.

How do I overcome irrational fear memories that continue to be triggered even though I might know, rationally, that I am safe?

We trick, or rewrite, our memory.

Building a Chilled Memory

The key to rewriting a memory is accessing it. It is hard to bring up a file on your computer if you haven't turned it on. Suppose the memory had emotion in it, such as fear. In that case, we need to access the memory enough to evoke the feeling. If we don't access the emotion, we haven't brought up the file we need to change.

That is why rationally saying that being afraid of spiders is stupid doesn't make our fear of them disappear. By being rational and not including the feelings, we aren't fully accessing the scenario – the file – behind the fear. As we've already seen, unless we change the scenario our brain uses to make us afraid in that circumstance, the fear remains.

This all may sound complicated, but ultimately the solution is simple. We often know it as desensitisation.

Dull Is Good

Desensitisation, in simple terms, means we create a calm or dull memory. No fear, please; we keep it boring.

There are several approaches to desensitising. Each approach requires us to trigger the fear, to be afraid. Then we learn to create a new memory by letting, or actively working to let, our fear pass – to be calm.

Some are very gung-ho with this. For example, if you are afraid of heights, they'll take you to the top of a tall building, and you stay there until you calm down. Once you are calm, you leave. They may do this several times until being up high isn't so scary for you anymore. Your brain has learned it is OK. They would use a similar approach for social anxiety, fear of spiders or snakes, or fear of public transport.

I prefer a gentler approach, also known as graduated desensitisation or graduated exposure therapy. Essentially, we reduce our fear a bit at a time.

Graduated Desensitisation

Consider the following example of how we might desensitise a fear of spiders.

Suppose even the thought of a spider terrifies you. We imagine we are in our safe place and are calm. Then we imagine the spider at the other end of a vast, empty warehouse. If we feel too scared to cope with that image, imagine the spider on the other side of town, locked up somewhere it can't get out. Then imagine the spider getting a bit closer. As that starts to scare you, hold that image and calm yourself by using a calming meditation like the Focus on the Breath mindfulness skill that we learned in Chapter 4. Hold the image of the spider until you are completely relaxed and calm, and then stop.

We do the same the next day.

We gradually bring the spider closer in our minds until we are OK with it being close and still feel calm. Then we stop and repeat.

Once we are calm with the image in our mind, we might look at pictures of spiders and learn to calm ourselves while looking at them.

Lastly, we expose ourselves to a tiny spider in a jar in the same room and calm ourselves down as we have already practised.

The critical part here is that at each stage in the process we leave feeling calm – bored – with no feelings of fear or distress, so we can use that as our new memory to build upon next time.

A similar form of desensitisation works for fear of heights, fear of flying and all other manner of phobias. But, again, if you need help, there are many therapists happy to take you step by step through this process.

There is no shame in seeking help. Overcoming some fear memories can be challenging. They can be very slow to shift.

Does desensitising myself to fear also use a plan or acceptance to resolve it?

Yes.

By creating a new way to react to the fear, we are rewriting our plan – what we will do. The new plan for the place or thing that triggers the fear is to be calm and practise our calming skills.

Staying next to what terrifies us and letting our fear reduce is like calling its bluff earlier. We accept it is there, and there is nothing we need to do to make a difference. The fear then settles and becomes our new, calm memory.

Try it. Set aside days to gradually expose yourself to places or objects you are afraid of – assuming they are safe. Sitting beside a live, big rattlesnake to cure a fear of snakes isn't what I'd call safe. If it was in a glass aquarium with a tight lid, no problem.

Always be safe.

Persist, and you will succeed.

*****

For Melinda, rehearsing success was the key, but ensuring she left work feeling calm also helped. By ensuring she had calm memories of work, she had less reason to worry when she entered the building for the next work shift.

*****

OK, this sounds good, but what if I have fears so powerful that I can't even begin to face or imagine them? What do I do then?

We use a gentler and less direct approach.

CHAPTER 13

ADDING JOY AND A TALE

Stage 3 continued

It is easy to see our problems and fears in a single way and hold onto that view no matter the consequences and how it makes us feel. But what if we began to see them differently?

Step 9. Create a Joyous New Picture

In the 2016 HBO series Westworld, we see a future where robots are made to be so much like humans that they become self-aware. But unfortunately, the robots are made to satisfy the carnal lusts of human beings and suffer terribly. Among the horrors, the main character, Dolores Abernathy, a sentient robot, offers a powerful and relevant quote: 'Some choose to see the ugliness in this world, the disarray. I choose to see the beauty. To believe there is an order to our days. A purpose.'

Even though this was a programmed response, Dolores reminds us that the story – the narrative – we live by determines how we feel. We can choose to see the horrors and be brought down by them or see the world differently and feel better for it, if even for a short time. The same is true for fears. If we choose to change the story around them, the fear can be tamed. Changing our stories to see the world differently is called reframing. Reframing is one of the most powerful tools we have for taming fears.

Why is it so powerful?

Because reframing completely rewrites the scenario that our brain is so afraid of and turns the events on its head.

We've already tried some reframing in the questions we asked our fear when we called its bluff. Here we can take the reframe to a whole new, more potent level.

The key to using reframing to tame a fear is flick the joy switch.

Joy Switch = Fear Dissolver

We all have a joy switch, a switch we can turn at a moment's notice to completely change what we see, to see it in a better – yet still realistic – light. We've already begun to use our joy switch.

Remember when we called fear's bluff when we were petrified our partner would leave? One of the questions we asked was, would breaking up and learning from the mistakes of this relationship set me up for an even better relationship in the future? Likewise, we wondered when facing the fear of losing our home whether we could rebuild, perhaps start anew – might end up with a better home.

In other words, would I still be afraid if I felt I would be better off rather than worse off if my worst-case fear came true?

Why be so afraid that we devise a plan to stop our partner from leaving, for example, if we feel we would be better for the relationship ending? Our brain is no longer frightened by that scenario.

And here is the key: we only get afraid if something important is under threat, such as losing something or someone important to us. If we see that we would be better off, there is no reason to be afraid. We aren't afraid.

Reframing isn't about turning a dirt sandwich into a peanut butter delight. It is about choosing to see the payoffs, the rewards, more than the losses. Some call this preferring to see the glass half full. Unfortunately, I don't think that analogy does justice to the power of reframing.

So, you know your fear and have named it. You have sat with it; the fear monster is looking at you in the face. Now, talk to it. 'You know, Mr Fear, there are many payoffs you might not have considered. What do you think about these?'

Once your fear monster sees the benefits are so much more valuable than any possible loss, it will likely shrink to a manageable size. Then, it will give you a hug and walk away.

One less fear. Bye!

Is it always easy to find the positives?

No, the brain will often go into threat and loss mode as it tries to motivate us to prevent a tragedy. And thoughts of an uncertain future won't help. The unknown is scary; our brain will want to avoid that. But with coaxing and some guidance, putting the effort in to see the benefits – turning on our joy switch not our threat switch – it is incredible what we can find.

Does reframing work to tame every fear?

No, but it can help.

Most importantly, reframing offers us hope and prevents us from feeling trapped. For instance, if we are so afraid of leaving our partner for fear of being alone that we accept their lack of love, we are trapping ourselves in a heartless relationship. Suppose we are so afraid to leave our job that we are overworked and underpaid. In that case, we are trapping ourselves in an unhealthy position. There is hope beyond a heartless relationship. There is hope beyond exploitation in our job.

Unless we see beyond the fear and reframe it to see the positives, our fear will trap us and prevent us from having a much freer life.

If you haven't already, let's try flicking the joy switch.

Look at any remaining fears from your list. Write down the fears below. Now, for each, write a list of positive alternative outcomes. Think of the ways the scenario you fear can work for you and not against you. Focus on as many positives as you can. Write down at least five.

Fear ....

Positives
1. ....
2. ....
3. ....
4. ....
5. ....

If you struggle to see the positives, think about what you might learn from the threat or loss. How can the experience prevent you from going through this again? What lessons would you share with others (such as your children) so they might also learn from this? Look beyond the fear and let yourself see the fear in a more realistic and positive light.

Reframing is particularly useful for taming the fear of failure.

Use the Joy Switch to Tame the Fear of Failure

As we've seen, learning to rehearse our success is a great way to overcome our fear of failure. But so too is reframing – using the joy switch.

When we are afraid of failure, our brain only focuses on the negatives, not the positives. It focuses on how we don't meet expectations, how others might be disappointed in us, how we let ourselves and others down or how we just don't live up to our own high standards. There is often tremendous pressure to be perfect and not make mistakes.

But that isn't a very useful or realistic story, is it?

A story that is closer to reality and more useful is to recognise we are made to make mistakes. Our brain is a refinement organ. It keeps learning and improving to get more effective and efficient. So how can we get better at anything if we never allow our brains to make mistakes?

Making mistakes is necessary. Mistakes are normal. Making mistakes can be very helpful – a good thing.

Our society punishes failure. No wonder we are afraid of it. But what if we learn to seek out failure to increase our chances of success? What if every failure is a learning opportunity that makes us better people and better at our relationships, jobs and life? What if failure is our tool and path to success? Flick the joy switch on a fear of failure, and what is there to fear?

The story we tell ourselves determines how we feel. Choose a different story, and we can tame innumerable fears.

But I can't see the good, the only images in my mind are horrible, and they won't stop. What do I do?

Have you ever heard the story of the good wolf and the bad wolf? It is a story I have heard before and seen in the movie Tomorrow Land, the 2015 time-travel movie with actor George Clooney. The story goes something like this – and I'm paraphrasing.

Inside each of us, it is told, there is a good wolf and a bad wolf. The good wolf makes us think good thoughts and do good things. The bad wolf makes us have bad thoughts and do bad things.

Which wolf wins? In other words, which wolf is stronger: the good wolf or the bad wolf?

It is the one you feed. If you give energy and attention to the bad wolf, you will have bad thoughts and do bad things. On the other hand, if you give your energy, focus and attention to the good wolf, it will be victorious.

It is the same with flicking the joy switch. You can choose to put your energy into thoughts and plans for good and positive outcomes about fear or to put your attention and energies into the bad outcomes. The latter will make the anxiety stronger. The former will make the fear monster leave you alone. It is your choice. The fears and thoughts have no special strengths or powers other than those we give them.

*****

OK, I've tried all this, but some fears are just too hard to face no matter how I try.

Some fears are so severe we try to forget them and often do. How do we tame these fears? We learn from a famous author.

Step 10. Harry Potter It

Have you heard of Joanne Rowling, born in 1965 in England? Maybe you know her under her better-known name: JK Rowling, the author behind the highly successful Harry Potter fantasy book and movie series. As a public figure, we have learned of her rags-to-riches story and her struggles with traumatic life events, especially in her teenage years and as a single mum. Life was tough. Rowling found an excellent way to help her cope, and to earn a living: she wrote about her problems through fictional characters on a page. It offered a detached way to explore, integrate and heal a part of her troubled self.

Art can be amazingly therapeutic in many forms, including dealing with our most potent and hard-to-face fears.

Suppose we have fears so deep and terrifying that we can't bear to consider them. In that case, trying to sit with them, call their bluff and rewrite them can seem impossible. Flicking the joy switch? Not going to happen.

That is OK.

Shutting ourselves away from severe traumatic memories is how we can still get by in life. It is better than collapsing in a heap every few minutes. But, if we seek to tame and resolve these more profound and most potent fears, stop the concerns from the past still haunting us, then it is often helpful to tame them in a roundabout way rather than head on. This is where art comes in.

How do we use art to tame fear? What can art do to help us resolve anxiety and find our plan or acceptance?

Consider the following.

Paint, Draw or Sculpt It

One way to get to know and rewrite a deep and hidden fear is to express the fear on canvas, on paper or in a 3D sculpture. Let it all out. Express what you feel in physical form, through drawing, painting, computer art, clay sculpture – whatever medium you like. Then, keep refining the piece until it feels right, until it represents something close to what your fear or trauma feels like.

Search for a representation of the fear – an image that gives it expression – but also for images representing its resolution, its transformation. It may take some time, but every instance you hold that image – that feeling – you are starting to recognise it, to name it. As you explore how to transform the feeling, you will rewrite it. And each time you access the fear as close as you can to when you first felt it, the more you become tolerant of it – accept it – and the less it continues to affect you.

Explore the qualities and characteristics of your fear. What parts of it are making you afraid? Then, paint, draw, sew or sculpt images reflecting this. Use colours and textures that feel right to you.

But I'm not an artist.

It makes no difference. You don't need to be a trained artist to do this. No one needs to see your work. These are works of expression and exploration from the heart. It is up to you what form they take.

Take your time.

If you want professional help to deal with your fears more profoundly and to experience the transformative potential of art, seek a trained art therapist.

Write About It

As we have seen, stories are powerful, even stories about fictional characters. If we write a story with honesty, from our hearts, then we grow and change ourselves. Write about our days and what we felt like, and we integrate our experiences and feelings into our life. A typical way to do this is to write a private diary or journal.

I like the approach of imagining we are writing to a friend overseas who we cannot see – no video calls. Any story written from the heart is therapy.

Does what I write have to be well thought out, have a plot, turning points, a proper climax, and resolution at the end?

No, not unless you intend to sell it, as JK Rowling did. The key to using writing to access and rewrite a fear that is too difficult to tackle head on is to write it for us alone, as if no audience would ever see it.

But I can't write.

That doesn't matter either. As you write and express your feelings, you automatically get better at it and find it easier; the words tend to come.

What do I write about?

If you are up to it, you can write about your life, how events made you feel and how they made you the person you are now. If that is too confronting, create fictional characters who have motivations you are familiar with, such as jealousy, anger and revenge. Explore why the characters do what they do based on your experiences of those feelings and what has made you who you are today. None of the characters must be exactly like you. That's the good part about writing: you choose how much you look at yourself as you write. If you want to write a fantasy where you have magical abilities like Harry Potter has, abilities that empower you so you feel less afraid, then do it.

I know some writers who find it therapeutic to create characters that remind them of people who have hurt them and make them suffer in the story they create; it gives the writer a form of release. If you need to include in your story a person or people like those who once traumatised you, and give them what they deserve, then feel free. Let it out. I know one writer who wrote a character who was the spitting image of a toxic ex. He killed her off early. Apparently, he felt better after it.

You are the author. It's your story, and you choose how you resolve your fears in it.

Write, and let it flow until you have it all out. Don't edit it. Don't go back over and over it to get it perfect.

Play or Dance It

Perhaps you are more musically inclined. Maybe you have started to play a musical instrument. Wonderful. We can use music to help us heal too. The key is to play what you feel, play notes or tunes on your instrument that express you. Don't worry about composition, beat or the usual music rules; break them. Express your heart in the sounds. Also express your healing and what that would sound like.

Contact a music therapist if you think you need help with this. Explore your feelings together.

You might prefer to explore your fear by using dance, to express it in your body's movements, to dance what you feel and let it out. Express the fear and feel where it is. Then feel the actions you need to take for the fear to be released. This isn't dancing for an audience; this is dancing to connect with you and to heal. Let it flow, unrestricted, without expectations.

*****

Head to the whiteboard now. Write it in; set in your art time. Art therapy time doesn't happen unless we make it happen, unless we realise its great potential and power and make it a priority.

*****

Did Melinda use art as therapy? She occasionally painted but she resolved her fears enough using the other steps we mentioned above. She didn't feel compelled to use art to assist a cure.

Melinda and her husband delighted in the arrival of their second child several months ago. Melinda is confident her children will not have to suffer the anxieties like those that temporarily incapacitated her. She has been off all medication for at least a year. Of course, we remain on the lookout for any relapses, but Melinda remains confident in her new fear-taming skills.

*****

Later we will tame Covid-related fears. Before we get to that, let's consolidate what we have learned in the following mini-workbook chapter. I suggest you copy the pages of the next chapter to use for any unresolved fears you still have and for any that arise in the future. Following the mini-workbook chapter, we will try using our new fear-taming skills to tame fears related to illness and death.

CHAPTER 14

MINI-WORKBOOK

This chapter is both a summary and a set of practical steps derived from what we have learned to tame, or resolve, a fear. When helping a client tame a fear, I wouldn't necessarily use all the steps; often only a few are required. It isn't practical to include a set of steps tailored to your unique needs. Instead, I have included all the steps.

I would recommend trying each of the steps in order. Some may be more relevant and helpful than others. I suggest you let your instincts guide you to which steps you want to focus your attention on most. Don't just try the easy steps if your gut says the more challenging steps will benefit you most. Having said that, all the skills can be useful at some time or other with one or more fears. It is helpful to have many tools in our tool chest.

Reminder: Fear Secrets

We begin with a reminder of some critical secrets of fear we can use to help master it:

- Fear is a natural human response; it is our friend.
- Fear only exists when our brain looks to the future.

- We are made to be afraid of the unfamiliar; being afraid of the unknown is normal.
- We become afraid when our brain runs a dream, story or fantasy simulation of the future.
- Fear can be resolved; we can make it go away.
- Our brain will keep bothering us with fear until we give it a plan and/or acceptance.

Ways to Reduce Our Fear Burden

Behind each individual fear is a significant burden of fears restricting our lives. While this fear burden can make it more challenging to resolve – tame – our individual fears, there are several ways we can reduce it.

Box It: Compartmentalise

We don't let work problems disturb us in our social times and vice versa. Have you bought your worry book yet?

Use Mind-chill Skills

Mindfulness meditations are a powerful way to calm and train the mind. Which of the four do you practise and prefer? Can you now switch off your thoughts when you need to?

Shift from Busy to Happy, Manageable and Chilled

If we are too busy we won't deal effectively with our fears. It is helpful to use a list of life priorities to guide where we can cut back. Are you living your life in line with your priorities? Are you taking the time to make time?

Find Peace in the Predictable
Our brain finds peace in the predictability of routine and structure. So how is the whiteboard going? What about your functional habits and traditions? Have you adopted or changed any of these?

Find Peace in Connection
The more predictable people are, the less afraid of them we need to be. This means building social connections. Have you found, or started to build, your tribe despite the challenges of Covid?

Dial Down the Scary Stuff
The media can scare us far more than we need to let it. It can be hard to cut back on watching the media. Do you search out many sources of information rather than believe only one view? Have you started more respectful conversations founded on sharing news rather than proving you are right?

Tap into Nature's Peace
It is easy to lose sight of our place in the natural world and get caught up trying to keep up with the Joneses. Nature offers us a way to slow down, to match its slower rhythm and connect with a more significant part of ourselves. How often do you connect with the part of nature that best soothes and centres you?

Importance of Reducing Our Fear Burden
As we have seen, when we reduce our fear burden, we can often resolve many individual fears too. One example is finding peace in connection, which can tame many social anxieties. As we can now see, taming

fear isn't just about finding what we are afraid of and resolving it; it is also critical to resolve our overall fear burden.

With our fear burden down, we are in a better place to resolve our troubling individual fear.

10 Steps to Resolve Your Fear

Step 1. Find a Safe Place

Name and describe your physically safe place.

> **My physically safe place is**
> ....
>
> **What makes it safe?**
> It is safe because [I have added a few examples]
>
> 1. No one disturbs me.
> 2. I can escape here whenever I need to.
> 3. ....
> 4. ....
> 5. ....

By listing why our chosen physical place is safe, we can be more confident it is as safe as we need.

*****

Name and describe your mentally safe place.

My mentally safe place is
....

Describe your mentally safe place.
My mentally safe place looks like
....

In my mentally safe place, I feel
....

Describe five features of your mentally safe place, such as the appearance of any plants you can see. Describing details helps consolidate the place in our mind, making it more precise. This makes it more accessible when we need it.
Five features of my mentally safe place

1. ....
2. ....
3. ....
4. ....
5. ....

Remember, if we finish a session of trying to tame fear and the fear hasn't been settled or resolved, we will end our session in this mentally safe place.

Step 2. Name It to Tame It

Only you can know what you are afraid of.

Don't let anyone tell you what your fear is. Don't make fears and memories that don't exist because you think they must be there or someone tells you they are.

Avoid denying a fear out of ego or pride. It is OK to be afraid; it doesn't lessen us.

Don't judge your fear as either good or evil. Fears are just a response, neither good nor bad.

Now I would like you to draw your fear – what it looks like for you. Give your fear – your balloon monster – whatever name you like. I call my fear Cade, for Can't Actually Do Anything. Here is Cade: my balloon monster.

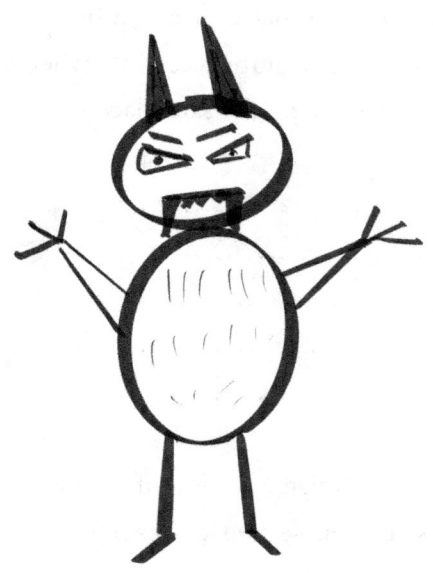

CADE

Remember, drawing can help us process our fear from a safer and more manageable distance. It is therapeutic.

Try drawing. What have you to lose?

As you can see, I can't draw either.

What fear does your balloon monster represent? Write it below.

My fear is

....

Step 3. Reality-check the Fairies and Unicorns

You will recall our brain is a great fantasy maker. Its worst cases are fantasies, and many of them are ridiculous. Let's see if your fear is realistic enough to bother with or waste your time and energy by answering the following questions.

What is the chance of your fear actually/realistically happening? Mark it on the line below: 0% to 100% likely.

0% _____100%

So, is your fear realistic? (Circle one.)

YES   NO

I can imagine five jumbo jets crashing over my house at the same time in the next week. Does that mean I should move? Likely chance of it happening = 0% or close enough. Is the fear realistic = NO.

Is your balloon monster still there?

Yes?

Then we continue.

Step 4. Have a Sit-down

Draw yourself seated in a room with your balloon monster sitting in a chair opposite. I have drawn an example. The room and the figures can be huge or small; it is up to you. You might like to draw yourself being larger, more significant, than the balloon monster. You can make the monster small, represented by them being a long way away.

Draw one speaking bubble above you and one above the monster. Write in each bubble the word HELLO! I'm shouting because they might be a long way away.

Wave to each other in the diagram if you like.

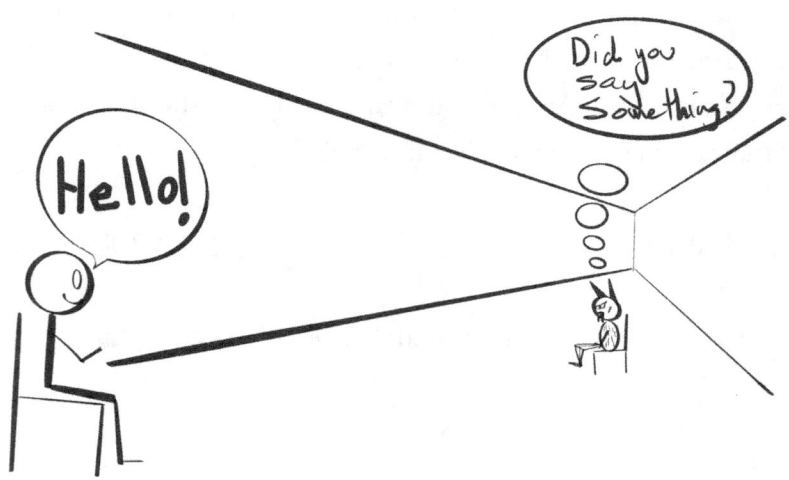

Imagine you are in that room with your fear. Sit with it. Say hello again. Wave to it again. Hi.

Just sit and imagine getting used to each other's company. Whatever you do, don't let them get up and leave. Tie them to the chair if you have to. Hold the fear there so you can chat.

Step 5. Have the Chat and Ask the Primary Question

Draw you and your balloon monster sitting closer together, facing each other. Next, draw a speech bubble above both you and the monster, and in your bubble, write: What do you want from me to go away?

Then, fill in the balloon monster's reply if you know the answer. Make sure the solution is realistic; no superpowers accepted. No, the solution to bullying is not to be Thor, God of thunder.

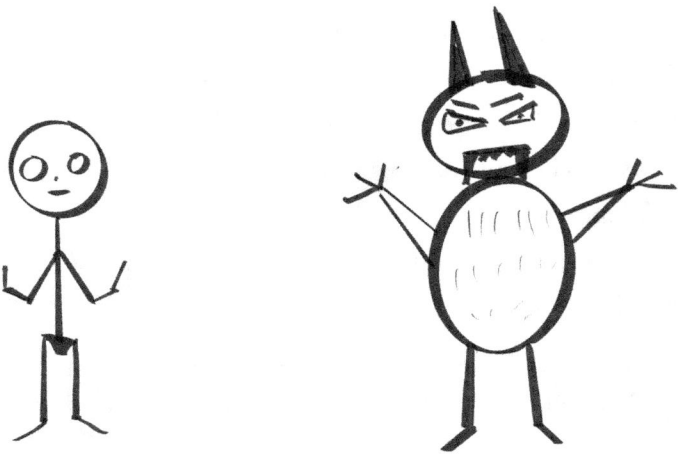

Think about the realistic solution your balloon monster gave you. Is it a solution you can act on? (Circle one.)

YES   NO

If it is a solution you can act on, list what steps that might need you to take.

To resolve my fear, I can

1. ....
2. ....
3. ....
4. ....

Remember, all our balloon monster wants to know is our plan – what we will do – or see that we accept that there is nothing we can do that will make a difference. If we have a list of what to do and can commit to it, great. It may be as simple as studying for an exam, being better prepared or doing some research to know what we're up against. Whatever it is, we put it on our list. We commit to it, so our brain knows it will be OK. If we can't commit, we aren't giving it much confidence, are we?

If we don't have a list, or have a list but one we can't commit to, what do we do?

We ask the monster another question.

Ask your balloon monster: can you accept that nothing I can do will make a difference?

Does your monster agree and realise there is nothing you can do? (Circle one.)

YES   NO

If the answer is no, we can expect the fear monster to still be sitting there waiting for your plan – the solution. So, we either give the fear monster what it needs, or it hangs around like a bad smell and remains big and scary.

> **CRITICAL POINT**
>
> Whenever a new fear shows up, ask it the question: what can I do to make you go away?
>
> Then ask the following question: can you accept there is nothing I can do to make a difference?

Is your giant and scary-looking balloon fear monster still there?

Yes?

Then we call its bluff.

Step 6. Call Fear's Bluff

Calling our fear's bluff can be a shortcut to resolving it. We can take one of two approaches: we can be direct and let the fear give us its best shot or we can be indirect and explore it from the inside.

We will initially consider the direct approach, should you wish to try this first.

The direct approach, as we described, means letting the balloon monster blast at us full on – giving us its worst until it is tuckered out.

It means we have to stand our ground. We can't pull out at any time, or we are back where we started.

It means summoning a bit of courage.

It also means taking my word for it, that no matter how intense fear is, no matter how horrid it makes us feel, it is all bark with no bite; it truly is a balloon monster, full of hot air. Yes, the feelings the fear will bring up when we fully confront the fear will be intense and make us terribly uncomfortable. Fear naturally does that. But the intensity can't – and doesn't – last.

If we commit to this, the key is not holding back or stopping too soon.

We do not attempt this method to resolve a fear if we are not prepared to see it through, as that can discourage us.

If we can't see it through, instead we step inside the fear and look around – the less direct approach. We keep persisting with our explorations. Know the inside of the fear well, and it will fade.

Shall we give the direct approach a try?

Direct Approach

Draw the following. You are standing face to face with your fear: the balloon monster. You are so close it starts to terrify you. Draw the monster shouting and getting angry, arms in the air, much bigger than you.

Now, close your eyes and let the fear walk through you like a ghost, in all its rage, aggression and frustration. Let it lose all control. You just stand there, still. Don't try to calm it. Don't try to understand it. Don't try to reason with it. Let the fear be free to go off inside us unrestricted.

It might take seconds, it sometimes takes a few minutes, but the fear can't keep up this level of intensity. If we have truly let it give us its worst, fully imagined, the worst fear coming true and all that feels like, then it will pass through and come out the other side of us. It has taken any remnants of it with it.

Don't forget, if we hold back even a little and not let us feel the fulness of the fear in all its intensity, it is like it leaves something inside us.

Remember, it is just a fear – a scenario of your brain you are facing, a possible future. The fear will simply create a physical reaction inside you. Let it. You are in a safe place.

Give it a try.

How do you feel?

If you feel the fear is gone – is resolved, like a weight lifted from your shoulders – then draw a picture of you, tall and strong. Then, beside you draw the small, soft and diminished monster that can only make a barely audible squeak.

Well done.

If you didn't succeed, you can try again or leave it for another time. If you leave it for another session, I highly recommend you go to your mentally safe place and be there for at least several minutes because the fear has now been woken. It may trigger bad dreams as your brain tries to find a solution on its own. This isn't necessarily a bad thing – unless you miss out on too much sleep and have to work the next day.

I often find the best fears to face and resolve are from my dreams or nightmares. Mind you, I rarely have any nightmares or severely disturbing dreams anymore. I find the fears from the night before are easiest to access during that day and hold onto. I'm happy to keep coming back to it as often as I need to until I resolve it. Often many memories and fears from my past show up. It gives me an excellent opportunity to understand them and the people who helped create them. Then, one by one, they disappear or become so insignificant I hardly remember them.

Draw your success and what that looks like. In other words, draw your fear when it is fully tamed. Please take the time. It helps reinforce the positives you have just experienced. It stabilises your new fear-free neural pathways.

If the direct approach isn't your thing, try the indirect approach.

Indirect Approach

Draw your balloon fear monster again standing in front of you – face to face. Imagine it is standing right in front of you. You know it is close because it makes you nervous or uncomfortable; the fear rises. Let the fear increase. That is good. Now we call its bluff in a way it doesn't expect.

Draw your fear monster again. Now draw inside it a representation of you in the monster. You haven't been eaten; you are inside looking around. Imagine the surprised look on its face. Draw that too. I bet it didn't see that coming. We've never done that before.

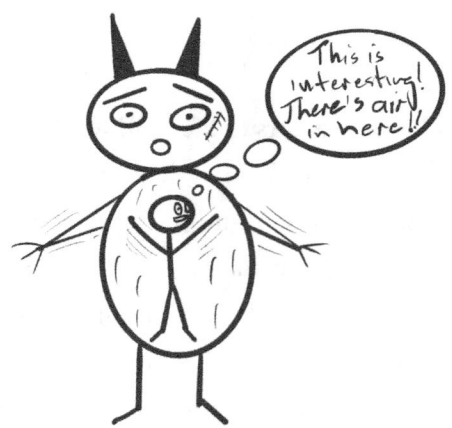

Now you are inside it, write a list of questions you'd like to ask it. As you ask each question, feel how it responds. Notice what changes within the fear.

I'll get the ball rolling.

1. Will I still be worried about you in five or ten years?
2. If the worst case happens, will the people I cherish most still be there for me?
3. Am I putting all my eggs in one basket when ultimately it probably won't be that important?
4. Can I pick myself up and do better if the worst case happens?
5. Who taught me – created – this fear? Are you a childhood fear I still need to be afraid of?
6. Are you made up of other fears? Is there more than one?

Be curious. Write any questions that will help you see the fear in a new light or better help you to understand where it came from and why it bothers you. There are no silly questions.

The more we ask the fear and search for honest answers while we are inside it, the more we rewrite it in our brains; we change it and tame it. We also get used to it, which helps it fade.

Another powerful question to ask your fear is, was it my fault? Have a look into your past, the memory or scenario that triggered the fear. Ask the fear: was it my fault or did it happen because of others and how they treated me? Did I do the best I could at the time? You will recall how I overcame many fears related to schoolyard bullying by questioning from within the fear.

Take your time.

Persist. Come back to the same fear if it is still there; often it will be and it can last for some days or weeks or more. Explore inside it. What we want is inside our fear, not outside looking in. Imagine your worst fear comes true, now what? Draw the monster anew each time you explore it.

Do you still have fears you struggle with?

Yes.

Let's apply some supplementary skills.

Step 7. Rehearse Success: Simulator Magic

We know if we imagine failure, we feel afraid. Imagining failure makes it more likely since we are rehearsing it in our brain – creating a memory of the future – for our brain to use for that event.

Better to rehearse how it will go well – to rehearse success.

How do I rehearse success?

1. Write down the outcome you are afraid of.

   I am afraid the following will happen
   ....

2. Write down what success looks like.

   Success for me means
   ....

3. Rehearse the physical steps – realistically – of what success looks like, of you succeeding. Then, keep repeating it over and over in your mind.
4. Every time the fear of failure comes up, replace it with the image and feeling of success.

If you are still afraid of failing, look at the bigger picture. Have you put all your eggs in one basket; are you letting this one event define who you are? If failure becomes only a small part of our lives, fear diminishes.

How do I deal with fears that make no sense, such as phobias?

We can use the next skill.

Step 8. Combat Memory Shenanigans

We can learn many fears from our parents and others around us. There may be no real reason to be scared now, but we have learned to be afraid, so our fear remains. We reduce these fears by creating calmer memories of the place or thing, such as spiders. The process we use to do that is called desensitisation.

Graduated Desensitisation

Draw your phobia or the place you are afraid of. Give it some detail, so it evokes images and feelings of fear; we want to access your brain's fear scenario/s. Now draw yourself a long way from that fear. When you finish drawing, do some simple breathing exercises to calm you like those in Chapter 4.

Me   **My phobia or fear**

On other pieces of paper, draw yourself getting closer and closer to your phobia or location. With each successive drawing, imagine you are getting closer. End each drawing with you being calm – chilled.

Finally, expose yourself to the real thing or place you are afraid of, starting by being far away then getting closer – like you did with your drawings. Each time you get closer, make sure you are calm, then leave. Get professional help if you are struggling.

Set aside a day in your weekly calendar or whiteboard devoted to desensitising you from a fear that annoys you and that you finally want to be rid of.

Once you have succeeded in taming this fear, draw a picture of what success looks like for you. It may be holding a spider in a jar, for instance, if you are afraid of spiders. It might be standing in a room that has terrified you or on a plane for the first time.

Congratulations.

*****

What about fears so powerful I can't imagine facing them? Or maybe I find the other methods too time-consuming, and they aren't suitable for taming the fear I have in mind.

Here are some alternative fear-taming skills.

Step 9. Create a Joyous New Picture

Reframing is a powerful tool to tame fears as it changes the narrative that has made us so afraid.

When our brain sees more positives than negatives in the predictive simulation of the future, then the fear dissolves. We can call this focusing on the positive as reframing and turning on the joy switch.

Joy switch = dissolved fear.

If you haven't already, write down your fear and then list five positives if the fear comes true: five payoffs.

Fear

....

Positives

1. ....
2. ....
3. ....
4. ....
5. ....

Think only of how this worst-case coming true will benefit you in the long run. We can all learn from the worst scenarios, assuming we survive.

Examples of typical positives include:

- I'm less likely to make the same mistake. I'll do it better next time.
- It wasn't my first choice, but it was my best choice in the end.
- I can use this experience and insight to make me a better person.
- I can pass on what I learn to others, maybe my children or grandchildren.
- To overcome a challenge is more rewarding. It will give me greater satisfaction.
- I never see myself as a failure. I am a strong and determined learner.

- Fear is not my weakness. Instead, it is my challenge that I will conquer and tame.
- My relationship ending means I might find a much better relationship next time.
- Losing my job gives me the chance to refocus my career in a better direction.
- When circumstance takes a loved one from us, we appreciate the wondrous opportunity to have shared hearts and love with someone so special, if even for the briefest of moments. It also helps us value connection with those around us even more.

Whatever the negative you can imagine, imagine the opposite: a positive.

Remember the good wolf and bad wolf analogy? Only feed the good wolf. Only give focus and attention to the images and thoughts of the positives.

Every time a negative thought comes along, automatically replace it with a positive. Soon you will do this naturally, as many of us already do.

Finally, if we are too overwhelmed by our fear, we use art to tame it.

Step 10. Harry Potter It

We have already used art to help temper our fear by drawing our fear above. If you didn't draw it and it still bothers you, please take the time.

The fear can look as horrible as you like. I have seen drawings with fire, knives and all sorts of horrid images. If that is your fear, let it loose on the page.

Now, beside the image of your fear monster or image, draw what it would look like if it were tamed.

My fear untamed   **My fear tamed**

How are the images different? What makes them different?

Perhaps you can draw what you can do to make that difference.

The final image I'd like you to draw is you walking with your tamed balloon fear monster, hand in hand, each of you with a pleasant smile on your face, as friends.

You have both been through a rough time. Unfortunately, the lack of communication has led to some horrible feelings and exchanges. But in the end, your fear monster only ever had your best interests at heart.

* * * * *

If you still need to communicate with your fear with a painting, sculpture, song, music, or dance, take your time and let it out of your mind and into the physical world; give it a physical form.

Always create a counter-image or sculpture of the fear tamed so your mind can also explore the alternative and get that image and all its feelings out too.

Remember, the art – the story, picture, sculpture, song or dance – you choose is for you and no one else to see or hear unless you let them. The art is there to help you communicate with a deeper you, and part of that deeper you are your fears.

Don't be embarrassed to seek out art and music therapists if available in your area.

How did you go?

Feel free to start again. But like we noted, fears can take more than one or two attempts to be tamed. Don't be discouraged.

Once you've tamed one often the next ones will be easier to tame. You have already shown your brain what it needs to do.

*****

To help us practise taming specific fears, let us see how we might apply the 10 steps to the fear of getting severely ill and the fear of death.

CHAPTER 15

NO, IT'S NOT A TUMOUR! TAMING FEAR OF SEVERE ILLNESS

'**D**oc, I've got this chest pain.' If you want to see a doctor's fear levels go up a few notches, it's all you need to say. Immediately, the doctor makes sure it isn't a heart attack; a blocked coronary artery can be life-threatening in moments. The problem was that Ken showed up at emergency around once every two weeks with minor chest symptoms he was convinced were a heart attack – or worse – and they weren't. Ken was an intelligent, rational guy in his early thirties, married, with no children and a well-paying finance job. He had no risk factors for heart disease, such as diabetes, smoking, family history or high cholesterol. The emergency would do all the appropriate tests then send him back to his regular doctor; it wasn't me. Each time the diagnosis was anxiety. For several years he suffered a near constant state of nervous tension that affected his sleep, at times preventing him from going to work. And he was annoying the heck out of his wife. No matter how many tests, he was convinced the doctors were missing some severe illness.

By the time I saw him, he was desperate. So far, none of the regular treatments for his anxiety had worked, neither medication nor counselling. The uncontrollable fear was getting Ken down.

Being scared to get sick is normal; no one wants to suffer unnecessary pain, misery or discomfort, or die prematurely from a terminal disease. A healthy fear of getting sick can make us look after ourselves and seek medical help early. However, Ken's fear of getting sick was no longer healthy. His fear was manifesting as physical symptoms, and the symptoms were real and bothersome. It's just that there wasn't a physical illness causing them. It was anxiety – fear. When a healthy fear of falling ill gets in the way of living, then, Houston, we have a problem.

Have you ever met someone who thinks they have every illness going around? I'm sure I have MS. It has to be rheumatic fever. I swear it's smallpox. But smallpox hasn't been around for decades! It doesn't matter, I'm sure I have it! So, what name do we often call these illness-focused and worried souls? Hypochondriacs.

Was Ken being a hypochondriac? Yes. Is labelling him as a hypochondriac helpful? No. It was essential to realise that he had illness-related fears, which needed to be resolved. The label wasn't going to help us tame his fear.

Fear surrounding having an illness can take many forms. It could be a fear of how the disease will lead to pain or suffering. It could be a fear of its impact on others around us. We may be afraid of dying before our time; we will look at the fear of dying more in a moment. No matter the fear, the basic principles to resolve it remain the same.

Interestingly, one of Ken's greatest fears was that illness would rob him of having a 'normal' life. He kept saying, I just want to be normal again. He was worried the condition would prevent him from working, having a family and living life to the full. The problem was, the more he worried about how the illness might take away from his life, the more it did; the fear was becoming a self-fulfilling prophecy.

Do you, or someone you know, suffer from fear – or fears – around having an illness?

Let us see how using the 10 steps to resolve fears can help.

10 Steps to Resolving a Fear of Illness

We begin as we have for resolving all fears: with preparation.

Step 1. Find a Safe Place

Before we face any fear, especially strong and influential ones, we must ensure we are in our physically safe place. Similarly, we must be familiar with our mentally safe place. We don't want to be disturbed, and we want to step back and calm ourselves if we need to.

Don't forget, if your fear becomes too much for you, please stop, take a breather, and rest in your mentally safe place until you settle. If that happens, try resolving this fear on another day. If, as is the case for Ken, the fear has remained for several years, then I'm sure it will still be there tomorrow; it won't be hard to find.

Step 2. Name It to Tame It

With so many types of fears surrounding illness, naming the fear is critical; we need to know what it is precisely about the disease we are afraid of. We need to be specific. Ken's main fear, as we saw, was the illness would rob him of his life, take away all that he treasured, take away hope. What does your fear threaten you with?

Remember, every fear is created by our brain running a simulation. So, what is your brain's worst-case simulation? What is it trying to get you to sort out?

If we struggle to work out exactly what the fear is, we often benefit from asking ourselves questions to probe the fear. Consider the following questions:

- If there was no pain involved, would I still be afraid?
- If there was no suffering of any type, would I be afraid?
- Have I seen someone else suffer badly from an illness that now scares me?
- Am I afraid of dying before my time?
- Am I afraid of the suffering I will put others through who have to care for me?
- Am I scared the illness will rob me of my dream life?
- Would I still be afraid if I could live my ideal life despite the illness?
- Am I afraid that if I get sick others will abandon me?
- Am I afraid of being severely disabled and reliant on others to get by?

The questions offer your brain scenarios to run through its simulator and develop feelings in response. By imagining removing what we might be afraid of, such as pain or suffering, we see if fear of these plays a role; would the fear still be there? If, like Ken, our fear is what effect the illness will have on our life, then what is our problem? After all, many people have terrible illnesses and can get the most out of what they have and cherish it, so why can't we?

I recall an inspiring fellow – Gerard – in his early forties, hunched over, unable to stand straight, his joints mangled, his fingers pointing where they shouldn't. He had many organs failing, all due to severe rheumatoid arthritis; this is before newer successful treatments were available. He loved cooking; perhaps it was his French heritage. He was motivated to be a good father to his teenage son. For him, every day was a bonus. Every time I saw him, he had a genuine smile on his face; it was another day to enjoy, despite the agony. He even smiled on the days he was in a wheelchair – the days the joints were too painful for him to walk. Oh, he'd occasionally grimace with pain, but he would tell a joke or anecdote and feel better for it. Gerard wasn't afraid of his illness or having a worse one, for reasons that would be obvious in a moment.

Do you know what precisely about the illness, or illnesses, you are afraid of?

Question your fear, run scenarios in your mind and see what creates your most significant fear response. Somewhere within that fearful image you made is the fear that grips you.

Once you know your fear, write it down here:

My fear is
....

If the fear is extreme and brutal to face, then I recommend you draw it and name it, as we did before.

If your fear is dying, we will consider taming that in the next chapter.

Step 3. Reality-check the Fairies and Unicorns

Oh, no, I have a pain behind my eye; it must be a brain tumour! It's a fever, it must be yellow fever, or a blood cancer – leukemia! My chest hurts, I must have myocarditis; I'm going to need a heart transplant for sure!

Good old Dr Google is scaring too many of us; a little knowledge can be a dangerous and scary thing. If we consider ourselves intelligent, it can make our problem worse. By looking up information on the internet, we become confident we are right, even though we have no clinical – real-world – experience of diagnosing or treating medical conditions. Soon we can create whole, seemingly realistic, fantasies about an illness we think we have or might get. Many exotic diseases can scare us.

The fear of illness is filled with fairies and unicorns, complete fantasies that can grab our attention and hold on tight.

The fear that we have, or may get, an illness needs a reality check. Often our fears are entirely bogus.

For example, most pains behind the eye are caused by headaches or other benign conditions NOT a brain tumour; a brain tumour behind the eye is extremely rare and often has different symptoms. Likewise, we can't have yellow fever if we haven't travelled to a place with mosquitoes that transmit it. And, yes, myocarditis – inflammation of the heart – is real. However, it is a rare side effect of the messenger RNA Covid vaccines. Still, the type of inflammation the vaccines cause does not lead to heart transplants; it is a mild, temporary condition. Besides, our new heart medications have enormously reduced the need for heart transplants.

Don't let the fairies and unicorns take you for a ride.

What is the best way to reality test whether the fear of having or contracting an illness is realistic?

First, find a medical professional you trust. Maybe see a few for a second or third opinion and let them share their knowledge and experience.

But doctors can get diagnoses wrong.

Yes, they can, and if you – unlike Ken – are usually rational and sensible about treating illness (you have no anxiety about it) and have a feeling – intuition – there is something wrong, then, by all means keep searching. But if you suffer a severe fear of the illness, I can guarantee you do not have a realistic view. In that case, we need to stop researching online and instead visit our GP to find out how real our fears are.

Step 4. Have a Sit-down

The stronger the fear, the more we need to learn to just sit with it. If the fear is too intense, draw you and your fear, as we did before. Draw yourself in a big room and the fear sitting far away. Eventually, you are sitting face to face.

Don't forget to say hello to your fear.

Whatever you do, don't avoid the fear or let it escape. Just share the space together. Practise your breathing exercise (see Chapter 4) if you need to.

Step 5. Have the Chat and Ask the Primary Question

Now you have the fear in front of you, ask the question: what do you need from me for you to go away?

If you are clear about what the fear of illness means for you, the answer may already be in your face. Perhaps, the answer is as simple as having a regular check-up with your family doctor.

If your fear has a solution, write down what you can do.

To resolve my fear, I can:
1. ....
2. ....
3. ....
4. ....

Put in place the plan it wants from you. Then, commit to it, as Anne did every morning when she asked herself what the fear needed from her for it to go away.

What if there is nothing I can do that will make a difference? Then we work on acceptance.

Acceptance

Why was Gerard not afraid of illness or even death? Why was he so appreciative of living? The main reason: acceptance.

Gerard had accepted there was only so much he could do with the crippling illness he had. His acceptance meant he wasn't comparing himself to how he could be and getting disappointed or sad because of it. Gerard wasn't building hopes of a cure and then being let down. He wasn't focusing on the parts of life the illness was robbing him of enjoying as much as accepting the joy that was still available to him.

Although Gerard only lived a few more years – he succumbed to his autoimmune disease – I know he made the most of it. I also know his son sincerely appreciated everything his father tried to do for him.

Don't forget, when you chat with your fear, ask if it is ready to accept there is nothing more you can do?

Well, fear, is there nothing more I can reasonably do? Yes? No?

I mean, there is always something more I can do, right? But is it reasonable? Can I accept that I don't need to do more than I am?

For instance, are these unproven and expensive treatments really worth it? Are they giving me false hope and making me feel worse for it?

Once we accept that we can't do much more than live a healthy life and have regular check-ups, once we follow the best advice available, then many fears of illness fade away. Realistically, in the end there isn't much more we can do.

Once our plans are being acted on or our acceptance realised, then our fear will settle; it will be tamed.

If our fear isn't tamed by now, we continue to step 6.

Step 6. Call Fear's Bluff

OK, so you get the illness you are so terrified of getting, now what?

As you will recall, there are two main ways to call a fear's bluff: a direct or indirect approach.

Direct Approach

Are you ready and willing to let the fear give you its worst? Are you ready to not hold back and instead let the ghost of your fear wear itself out inside you – let it have its tantrum and fade?

If you are, now is the time. First, follow the steps outlined previously in Chapter 11.

If you aren't ready to be so direct, we try the indirect approach.

Indirect Approach

The worst case for our illness comes true. What is our plan?

To help our brain consider its options, we can ask it questions specific to dealing with our health and possible sickness.

Some questions we might ask are:

- When did this fear start, and what triggered it?
- Do I need more trusted information?
- Who do I trust to help and inform me?
- What treatment would I look for, and where would I get it?
- Who can help support me through this? Who can I call on?
- If the treatment fails, what is my next plan?
- What steps can I put in place to avoid unnecessary suffering, and who do I talk to about this?
- What will I still be able to do?
- What can I reasonably do to prevent the illness without going to extremes?
- Am I afraid of dying?
- Can I accept that there may be no cure?

Look inside your fear. Be curious. Try to help your brain get as complete and realistic a picture as possible about what it is afraid of rather than rely on unreliable hearsay and false hope. Look at what can be done and what can't, and be honest about it.

Challenge your fear, test its assumptions – what it is assuming will happen. Will I necessarily get sick? Will I necessarily suffer as much as I think? What can I do about it? And if there is nothing more that I can do, what am I looking for?

*****

What questions do you think would help you to better understand and resolve your fear? Write them down here.

1. ………………………………………………………………
2. ………………………………………………………………
3. ………………………………………………………………
4. ………………………………………………………………

Come back to the questions every day until the fear is resolved – tamed. You can change the questions if new ones come to mind. Find what works. Seek help at any time you feel you need it.

*****

Unfortunately, Ken didn't find calling his fear's bluff much help. All he could focus on was how badly things would go and what he would lose, and, in his mind, it was everything.

Caution: Beware of Denial

As we start to explore the reality of our illness or potential illness, the fear can get so severe that we can be led down a path of denial. I won't get sick. I don't have that sickness. The specialists don't know what they are talking about.

I know of one chap, a lawyer, who was so scared of needles that he'd say all the illnesses overseas are just a way for drug companies to make money. He wouldn't take any medications to prevent infection or get immunised. He was fortunate not to get seriously ill. Now, not surprisingly, he is claiming Covid doesn't exist. It certainly gets him out of a needle.

When our brain can't cope with fear, the fears can be shut down with denial, until we get so sick the denial doesn't work or we die. Unfortunately, we have been seeing this with Covid. Tragically, people have been dying of the illness while denying it exists and is killing them.

If, on the other hand, we face our fear, get to know it, dissolve it on the inside, then we have a better chance of staying well.

Step 7. Rehearse Success: Simulator Magic

Ken couldn't help himself. All he could do was visualise getting worse – failure. So, we spoke about the good wolf and the bad wolf.

*****

Apply the step we learned to rehearse success earlier.

1. Write down the outcome you are afraid of.

I am afraid the following will happen

....

2. Write down what success looks like.

Success for me means

....

3. Rehearse the physical steps – realistically – of what success looks like, of you succeeding. Then, keep repeating it over and over in your mind.
4. Every time the fear of failure comes up, replace it with the image and feeling of success.

*****

Only we determine what thoughts or scenarios we devote our energies to. The thoughts only have the power we give them; there are no supernatural forces at work controlling us.

Ken related to the good wolf/bad wolf analogy, and his fears did start to lessen for a time. He would visualise his idea of success every morning and especially at night: how he would be, and would continue to be, well and physically what he needed to do to make it happen, such as regular walking, good sleep and a healthy diet.

If rehearsing success doesn't resolve our fear, we move on to step 8.

Step 8. Combat Memory Shenanigans

Bec hated doctors' examination beds with a passion. Bec was slim, intelligent and unmarried, with no dependents, and seemed naturally calm. Mental illnesses? She'd never had any, but ask her to even sit on the examination bed to look down her throat and her body tensed in obvious discomfort. She was terrified of the bed.

Why was she so afraid of the firm, vinyl-covered flat surface? You guessed it, a bad medical experience.

Bec had a terrible experience with the termination of an unexpected pregnancy several years earlier. Nothing about the procedure was explained, or she was too nervous about taking it in. There was no one to support her, and the pain and humiliation of the whole procedure left a horrible emotional scar.

Not all fears associated with illness are of an illness. Instead, as for Bec, it can be the procedures or other unknowns of the experience we fear the most.

Gradually, Bec and I built a rapport and spoke about the nature of fear. She found it very helpful to learn about the secrets of fear discussed earlier, so she knew what she was up against. Bec found it beneficial to know that her reaction was a natural response and that it wasn't her fault. It was also valuable to take her through how such a procedure might be better next time. Finally, we changed her memory of the event to feel differently about it, to not be so distressed.

This wasn't enough.

Eventually, Bec agreed to gradual desensitisation. Some of this was in the room getting closer to the bed. Most of it was her rehearsing in her mind being calm as she sat on and eventually lay back on the bed. This time she knew in her mind everything that would happen – no surprises. Little by little, her fear started to settle.

Three months later, she came in proudly telling me she'd had her pap test. A screening test for cervical cancer required her to lay on the bed as she had during the termination. Until now, she'd put it off due to her fear. Now her fear was tamed.

Are there any fears related to illness that you think will benefit from desensitisation? If so, write them here.

1. ....
2. ....
3. ....
4. ....

Take your time and work on desensitisation yourself. Of course, if you have any problems, don't forget to seek professional help.

* * * * *

Ken didn't find desensitisation helpful, so we tried reframing.

Step 9. Create a Joyous New Picture

As we have seen, when we are afraid, we are reacting more to what we might lose than what we might gain; fear doesn't exist if all we see are positive outcomes. Gerard was a great example of someone who focused on the positives of his illness.

Time to turn on your joy switch, like Gerard.

You have focused on what would go wrong and what your illness – or illness-related fear – will take from you. But, to be realistic, we also need to see the positives. So, I'd like you to name your fear again and then list the positives you could get from it coming true. Don't worry if you struggle at first to list any positives.

Fear

....

Positives

1. ....
2. ....
3. ....
4. ....
5. ....

Ask yourself what positive you could possibly have from your worst-case illness.

For example, perhaps you worry about cancer. What possible positives could you get from that? A cancer specialist I know had a great answer.

The specialist used radiation to successfully cure and treat many severe cancers; he'd seen some of the worst. He'd witnessed the suffering, the side effects of treatment and the anguish of the families. So, you would think he'd be the last person on the planet to want to ever have cancer. But he disagreed.

Cancer, the specialist said, would allow him to say his goodbyes and tie off loose threads. Better, he said, than dying on some random day by accident.

Yes, if I know that I will die in around two to three months, that gives me time to say what needs to be said, to leave life with a clear, unburdened heart.

I also find cancer gives us an excellent opportunity to live in the moment.

I recall many years ago a grandfather, Tony, with a close and supportive family, seeing me for depression and anxiety; depression and anxiety often go together. He was diagnosed with prostate cancer a few years previously. It was a minor, treatable type that wouldn't reduce his lifespan. Tony saw it differently. He believed the prostate cancer was killing him, and he was terrified of never seeing his family again. His fear and sadness were so bad he couldn't enjoy anything; he couldn't live.

After many discussions, Tony finally realised we could all die any time, so why not make the most of what we have left rather than worry about what we will lose? So, we called his fear's bluff and reframed it. We focused on the positives in front of his eyes, such as the precious time he still has with his grandchildren.

His life completely changed. With one change in mindset, Tony's family had back a happy, active grandfather with a new lease on life. He lived appreciating what he had. He was present in life again, making the most of what was there, like Gerard.

Illness has potential positives we rarely consider when we are well. For instance, it can help us reconsider our priorities to see who really cares, is important and is worthy of our time. It can trigger us to search for meaning and purpose and develop a deeper connection with our genuine selves. Illness can also offer us a chance to be kinder to ourselves and, importantly, remind us of our mortality and what that means for us.

Consider again the fear you have of illness. Now ask it: What can I get out of it that is worthwhile? How can it help me?

Maybe now you might find it easier to list the positives.

*****

Ken found the reframing helpful. He could see that overcoming this fear would give him skills to pass on to his children – give him confidence in his ability to face and overcome adversity, and better control his mind. He improved with a combination of rehearsal and reframing – using the joy switch. Occasionally he'd come back for reassurance, to be reminded of the power of the good wolf inside him. As a result, he is now a proud father and can engage with life rather than be trapped by worrying about it.

Step 10. Harry Potter It

Did you draw your fear monster of illness above? Have you written about your fear in your journal? Perhaps you have painted or sculpted your worst case and what the tamed version looks like?

If the other methods to tame your fear have not worked, now is the time to explore and tame it with art in whatever form you feel most connected to.

As you may have guessed, the writing of this book has been therapeutic for me; I find writing a book to be insightful and inspirational. I always learn something new about myself, others and the world. This is why I prefer to use the indirect approach for calling a fear's bluff; there is so much to learn about our mind, its priorities and the human condition. I wasn't always like this.

Throughout school and into university, I was heavily into maths, science and logic. Since the journey within in my twenties, I am now more focused and interested in feelings and learning how they affect what we experience and do.

What would you like to learn from understanding your fear, or fears, regarding illness or worries in general? What method of art might you prefer to explore?

No time like the present to start using art as your therapeutic tool.

*****

Ken tried some journalling. He wasn't into artful expression.

*****

In a world with so much information at our fingertips, it is easy to fear illness and everything associated with it, especially in the age of Covid. But, in the end, all our brain wants is to know what we can do about it and that we will be OK. So, take your time to fully understand your illness-associated fear. It can be a fantastic teacher.

* * * * *

So, was a fear of death one of your great fears associated with illness? If we are afraid of illness then we can expect that we will also fear death, especially if we are worried about severe illness. Resolving fear of death may seem like a futile or ridiculous task to some of us. Yet, how many of us are being manipulated and controlled by it? How many of us, like Ken, are prevented from living full and expansive lives thanks to our fear of dying?

To overcome a fear of death can have profound personal consequences.

We will use our 10 steps to help us finally tame this often-distressing fear.

CHAPTER 16

I'M GOING TO DIE!

Every time Dario, a fit young chap in his mid-twenties, suffered a stomach upset, his anxiety would go through the roof. This, of course, would worsen his stomach upset, and he'd be crippled with fear to the point he was sure of passing out, though he never did. He'd avoid restaurants and even family functions in fear of the terror that might afflict him. These symptoms had gone on for several months. We began to explore what the fear was about.

We faced his fear. He said he was afraid of vomiting or diarrhea. It had never terrified him before. It began when he was terribly sick with gastroenteritis several months ago. He needed to be admitted to the hospital for rehydration. But that wasn't the real fear. We explored further back.

It turned out that before these episodes started, he'd seen a good friend almost die from a stomach bug. Dario was by his mate's bedside in ICU and witnessed the suffering up close; no one was sure his mate would make it. After his close friend almost left this world, the thought that he might die from such an illness now terrified Dario.

Dario's greatest fear wasn't vomiting and getting diarrhea. Instead, he was afraid to die.

Every time Dario had the slightest stomach upset, he then thought this could be it; this could be the end. The fear of even the slightest stomach symptoms was now crippling his life.

Why tame my fear of dying? Isn't it a normal fear that keeps me alive?

Yes, our fear of death ensures we are careful and don't take stupid risks. Still, all too often, as was true for Dario, the fear of death can be so destructive in our life it can prevent us from truly living and can hold us back, as we saw with Tony a moment ago.

The fear of death is a perfect example of how critical the narrative, or story, we tell ourselves affects what we feel and what we do.

For example, recently I saw a young lady in her early twenties. She told me she was terrified of hell. She was so afraid of the possibility of eternal damnation she was unable to try new things without talking to her parents first. She was scared to have a relationship in case she made a mistake, knowing that marriage was forever. In addition, she limited her social connections to prevent hanging out with the wrong people. To her, hell was real. This belief was restricting her ability to develop an individual identity and was preventing her from trying life.

By contrast, for Anita Moorjani, the lady who claimed she'd died and returned, death makes life an incredible opportunity, one where we shouldn't be afraid to take risks. We should live life to its fullest and love each other and all things.

What we believe about death determines how we live, including how much fear we choose to live with.

Does the fear of death show up for everyone?

For many of us, the fear of death may not show up until we witness it or something happens to us to make us question, or come to recognise, our mortality. I have met several people who don't consider death at all – a denial and avoidance strategy. Others have become so obsessed with thoughts of death and mortality that it dominates their lives, causing fear and depression. Many of them have been in their early twenties. Not surprisingly, thoughts of death are bound to show up when illness is involved. One of our greatest fears of getting sick, as Dario found, was that we might die.

Mind you, Covid hasn't helped.

In the age of Covid, we often see the death numbers from Covid on our TVs or in the news feeds. Yes, we could get numb to it and put these numbers aside or we may reflect on them calmly. However, for some people, seeing the personal stories of death from Covid in their neighbourhood or region can trigger an enormous fear of dying – not just the fear of them dying but also the fear of losing loved ones. Will I be next? Will I ever see those I love again?

There are many reasons we fear death or are triggered into fearing death. As someone who has faced down and tamed the fears associated with our mortality (see the preface), I can confidently say that fear of death can be tamed no matter its cause. The fear of dying can be resolved.

We will now consider one approach to help us resolve our fear of death. We will be guided by the 10 steps outlined previously.

10 Steps to Resolving Fear of Death

Step 1. Find a Safe Place

By now, we will assume you have a safe physical place arranged, and a mentally safe place well-practised should your fear level get too high.

If your mentally safe place isn't easily accessible, now is an excellent time to go back and be sure you have a mentally safe place to retreat to should you need it.

Step 2. Name It to Tame It

As with many fears, the fear of death can have many components – many parts that make up the whole. Fearing death can be fearing losing what we cherish: fear of loss. We can be afraid of the unknown. We may fear a form of torment for our sins, such as eternal damnation. It could be the possible pain of suffering as we die or are about to perish. Some of us may fear the possibility there is nothing beyond life and, therefore, life has no meaning. To name the fear of death affecting you means distinguishing what is it about death – what scenario – you are specifically afraid of.

What particular part/s of dying are you afraid of? List them.

My fear of death is a fear of:
1. ....
2. ....
3. ....

Step 3. Reality-check the Fairies and Unicorns

Are my fears of death realistic? How can I know I am not making my fear up, and my worst fear isn't just a fantasy?

These questions can be challenging to answer. To help us make sense and answer them, let us break down the fear of death into two main parts:

- The fears are based on what we could lose from this life.
- The fears are based on what might happen after we die.

Let us consider each in turn.

Fears of Losses from this Life

Can we expect to lose physical things when we die?

The obvious answer is yes.

What can we lose when we die?

Everything. We will lose everything we own and have physical contact with, including everyone we know. Essentially, we will lose everything we have an emotional attachment and connection to. Imagine everything you cherish – gone.

It is not a fantasy to imagine enormous loss when we die. On the contrary, we are contemplating a genuine loss: the house, the car, the assets, the people are all lost to us. We can expect the brain to react to the threat of such total loss in three main ways:

a. It can react with sadness at the thought of the loss; perhaps feel depressed at the mere contemplation of it.
b. It can accept the loss and not feel much at all.
c. It can feel immense fear. It will put massive pressure on us to develop a plan to stop it from happening.

If you are afraid of what you may lose from life when you die, your brain is going with option c. Often, we have a mix of options a and c, with fear and feelings of sadness.

We will look at practical strategies to tame the fear of real loss in a moment.

Fears of What Might Happen After We Die

Considering our brain doesn't know what will happen after we die, its fantasy-prone brain can go nuts.

Unless you have survived a near-death experience, as Anita Moorjani claims, everything that we consider might happen after death is pure speculation – a creation of our mind; we haven't been to the other side to know. Yet, as we have seen, the stories and beliefs we hold about what happens when we die matter. They affect how we behave and act here and now.

In fact, our beliefs about death can profoundly impact how we live.

For instance, if we believe in karma, where the deeds of this life will determine how troubled our next life will be, we will want to be virtuous in this life to have a better next life. Similarly, suppose we believe in sin and punishment in eternal hell after dying. In that case, we may be less likely to do what is regarded as a sin, as was the case for the young woman mentioned a moment ago. Suppose we believe there is nothing after we die. In that case, we might focus on having a good time and not care about any of the rules that religions try to scare us into following.

We could also be so worked up about what we might have done wrong in this life that we become terrified to die. When death approaches, we are petrified – all thanks to a story we call a belief.

The fantasy, dream, belief or narrative we hold onto about life after death determines how we live and what we feel now.

And yet, ultimately, none of our stories or beliefs may be real or true; our mind has speculated.

When there is no way to reality test our ideas about the afterlife, we are at risk of coming up with the most outrageous possibilities. As we have seen, creating the worst cases is what our brain is made to do, and our brain has free reign when it comes to the hereafter. It can create anything it likes because there is no firm reality or proof to restrain it. Is it surprising, then, that so many of us are afraid to die when there are so many horrible worst cases running through our minds?

We will further consider how to tame such extreme fears related to death in the following steps. Suffice to say, if we can't prove it, we can be pretty confident there is a significant element of fantasy.

What category of the fear of death does your fear fall into? Is it realistic, founded on real loss? Or is it based in the less certain realm of fantasy?

Step 4. Have a Sit-down

If your fear of death is intense, then I recommend you draw a picture of it in a room with you, as before. Many cultures have images of death, from the Grim Reaper to Anubis, the Egyptian god of the afterlife. You may wish to choose one of those or make up one.

Eventually, draw you sitting in a chair opposite death.

Say hello. Wave.

Make space for fear. Hold the fear in your presence to ask it questions and get to know it.

Step 5. Have the Chat and Ask the Primary Question

Now you have your fear of death in front of you, ask it the primary question: what do you need from me for you to go away?

What image did it give you? Write down the answer.

Answer

....

Make sure your answer is both practical and realistic, that it can be implemented. Becoming immortal, for instance, is not a realistic solution.

Perhaps we see that we need to contemplate life and death more. Maybe we should make sure we follow the rules we believe in more diligently to ensure a better afterlife. On the other hand, we might need to reconsider our beliefs. Are we ready to consider alternative views that are less fear-based?

If we are fortunate, the fear may have answered us with the word 'acceptance.' Then we will know relief.

If our fear persists, we continue to step 6.

Step 6. Call Fear's Bluff

OK, so I die. Then what?

As we have seen, we have two main ways to call our fear's bluff: a direct approach and an indirect approach.

Direct Approach

Are you ready and willing to let the fear give you its worst? Are you ready to not hold back and instead, as I did, let the worst-case fear flow through you? Remember, my fear wasn't just of dying – I believed in life after death; what was at stake was my soul, my existence. If reincarnation existed, I was even prepared to sacrifice that. I did this out of necessity. I felt I had little choice.

You have a choice.

If you feel ready to face your fear of death and let it have its full tantrum so that it fades away, then what are we waiting for?

If you aren't ready, there is no shame.

Besides, you may gain interesting insights by peering inside your fear monster and looking around.

Should you choose this direct method, please follow the suggested process previously outlined.

Indirect Approach

We die. What is our plan?

We can break our options into two main parts to help our brain create an acceptable plan:

- There is nothing there. We no longer exist.
- We continue. Our consciousness, in whatever form, lives on.

To help clarify, let us add the two reality-test options we noted a moment ago.

- Fears of what we could lose from this life.
- Fears of what might happen after we die.

I know this sounds rather clinical; the fears and emotions we feel with loss and death are often deep, tragic and profound. For instance, I cannot imagine the pain and anguish a mother or father must feel leaving behind their children and grandchildren. I have no idea of the depth of heartbreak at the thought of losing our one trusted partner and companion we have grown closer to towards the end of life. I do not know the terror of someone who believes they are bound for damnation. However, overcoming my fears about death has given me some idea of what it is like to feel the latter.

The point is death is a topic filled with emotion. To help navigate these deep and difficult feelings, we can find it helpful to consider simple options. Considering these practical scenarios, we call fear's bluff by consciously allowing ourselves to see beyond the clouds of strong emotions. Then we can create realistic plans.

a. There Is Nothing After Death

What are our options if after our life there is nothing?

Can we still be afraid of the realistic prospect of significant loss? Definitely; perhaps now the stakes are even higher. There is no catching up with family on the other side. There is nothing to appreciate or experience once we are dead. The contrast between life and death becomes stark.

What can we do in response to potentially soothe our fear of such loss?

We can make sure we get the most out of life. We might work to prolong life. We can, like Gerard, learn to appreciate what we have and live more in the moment. Mind you, all these strategies prolong the inevitable.

Should we be afraid of pain and the sorrow of loss?

The only pain and sorrow we feel will be while we are alive. Once we are dead, we don't feel anything. So, there is nothing to fear on the other side.

The bottom line. Suppose we genuinely believe there is nothing after our life. In that case, ultimately, there is only one way to tame our fear of death: acceptance.

The best cure for fear of death when we don't believe in a hereafter is accepting our mortality; it's all going to end sometime. And when it does end, we have nothing to worry about. There will only be nothing.

b. Our Consciousness Lives On

How can we tame our fear of loss if we believe there is a hereafter?

We have several options.

For instance, if we believe in the afterlife, we can imagine our loss is only temporary.

Will we lose connection with those we love most when we die? Unfortunately, yes, but it will be temporary until, like Romeo and Juliet, we are together again on the other side.

Around twenty percent of people who die and then come back to life are able to recall their experience. Many, like Anita Moorjani in her book, *Dying to be Me* (Hay House Inc, New York, 2012), describe loved ones who have already passed are there to greet them.

To fill you in. Anita describes dying from the complications of incurable cancer. She was revived. On waking, she recalled that during her death experience, she saw her brother getting on a plane on the other side of the world. She recounted this before being told that he had in fact boarded that plane. Part of Anita's death experience was meeting passed loved ones and deciding to live. On revival, her cancer soon disappeared.

Belief in an afterlife can mean death isn't a permanent goodbye. Instead, it is a ciao, see you soon.

Can we still mourn the material items or privileges we had in life?

Sure. But if we recognise that these were only temporary anyway, they aren't so painful and scary to lose.

There is a truism: you can't take it with you. Everything we own or are attached to stays behind when we die. If, however, we value people most of all, then any loss isn't a loss, but like missing someone on a long holiday. Eventually, we meet again.

When there is no anticipation of loss, then there is no fear.

OK, but how do we tame fears about what might happen in the afterlife, like hell or eternal torment?

A nursing home nurse I see as a patient recently shared her view of death, having seen many people pass in her thirty-plus years of service. She said the people who deal best with death believe in something better on the other side. To her, it didn't matter what was actually there, if anything. What mattered most was what we believed, because what we believed affected how we felt here and now, among the living. What is on the other side, we will probably never know until it happens.

Her practical view has merit.

If our brain is fantasy prone and tends to create horrible worst cases that we know are ultimately not real, why not choose a fantasy or a story that works for you? Why not choose a story or belief that reduces fear rather than increases it and still gives our life meaning and purpose?

I am not here saying we must change our beliefs. Long and bloody wars have been fought to defend beliefs and impose them on others. All I am saying is by considering all our options and knowing the nature of our brain, we have ways to tame our fears of death here and now. Whether you choose to use them is up to you.

No matter our beliefs, we can always find comfort in acceptance. Even at the moment of our death, we can accept there is nothing more we can do.

As we learned from Tony with mild prostate cancer, acceptance is our choice. It is a shortcut to internal peace.

*****

> ## CRITICAL POINT
>
> There is a fear that if we believe in a pleasant afterlife and lose the fear of death, we will all want to get to the other side as soon as possible.
>
> That isn't necessarily true.
>
> For instance, Anita Moorjani, who believes in the pleasantness of the other side, also promotes life as a precious opportunity. Why? According to her experience of death, the afterlife is actually quite boring. We come here for the vivid life experience no matter how pleasant or painful; we chose this.
>
> Besides, it would be pointless to live just to hurry up and die to get to the other side. Our species would be extinct in no time! Obviously, there is more to life and death than meets the eye.
>
> Tragically, too many of us look to end our precious life experiences as a means of escape due to suffering. Yet, there are ways of changing how our brain sees itself and the world, so we don't feel bad. Perhaps now, more than any time in history, we are better positioned to learn the basics of what our brain needs to feel satisfied and live a fulfilling life. There is hope. If you have thoughts of ending your life, please seek help early.

When stepping inside the fear of death, there is much to explore and many profound personal insights to be gained. The key, as mentioned previously, is to be curious.

If our fear of death remains, we move to step 7.

Step 7. Rehearse Success: Simulator Magic

What would a good or pleasant death look like for you?

As we have seen, fear can often arise as we simulate – consider – our fai[lure]. But, of course, we don't want to fail, so our fear shows up and insists we de[velop] an alternative.

If you considered the best possible death experience or outcome for [you], would you still feel afraid?

Some of us are afraid we may suffer pain or discomfort in our last mom[ents]. Would rehearsing how we have excellent care and treatment remove that [fear]? Would having a quick death be a blessing? Would we still be as afraid if we k[new] we'd die in our sleep?

Apply the step we learned to rehearse success earlier.

1. Write down the outcome you are afraid of.

I am afraid the following will happen

....

2. Write down what success looks like.

Success for me means

....

3. In your mind, rehearse the realistic physical steps involved in that successful outcome. Imagine yourself succeeding. Keep repeating th[is] image over and over in your mind.
4. Every time the fear of a bad death experience arises, replace it with t[he] image and feeling of success you outlined above.

We may not know the circumstances or time of our death, but we can still rehearse and be prepared for it. The more rehearsal, the fewer unknowns. The fewer unknowns, the less fear.

Of course, the best rehearsal for death is to simulate acceptance – be at peace with what is happening and try not to fight it. The more we want to change the experience, the more fear will arise, and the more unpleasant the experience can be.

Try it. Rehearse truly accepting death and how it would make you feel.

Step 8. Combat Memory Shenanigans

Can we desensitise ourselves to the fear of death?

Sure, we can, but not necessarily in the way we might imagine.

I do not recommend experimenting and seeing how close to death we can go so we become tolerant to the fear. That is stupid. It is also dangerous and disrespectful of life. Those ideas can stay in the realms of Hollywood; they have made horror movies about such silliness.

On the other hand, we can desensitise ourselves to the fear by imagining it happening and then ensuring we are calm – by using our calming techniques. For instance, as we do our calm and focused breathing, we can tell ourselves repeatedly: I am OK, this is natural, I am alright. We hold the image we are afraid of and calm ourselves repeatedly. With a simple exercise like this, we rewire our brain so that thoughts of death have a different feeling than fear.

This is a similar method to rehearsing success but focuses more on settling remaining distressing thoughts about death.

If the fear doesn't go away, we can retry the other steps above or try step 9.

Step 9. Create a Joyous New Picture

There are always positives to see, even in our own death.

As we have seen, until we see the positives and the negatives, we aren't giving our brain a realistic picture to work with. So, instead, we restrict its ability to develop a plan or allow acceptance.

To help us consider some positives, consider the two main options noted above and flick the joy switch.

a. There Is Nothing After Death

If you believe no afterlife exists, can you think of any positives?

I can think of many. For instance, as mentioned, if we know there is no afterlife we can focus on getting the most out of the life we have – to be more appreciative, like Gerard.

If this life is all there is, why not work to make it the best experience possible? By realising we get our most profound satisfaction by helping others, for example, we are then motivated to make the world a better place and enjoy connection.

We have a greater sense of choice. We don't feel coerced by religions into doing what they demand of us. This means we can feel freer to choose what we do and why without the fear of afterlife torment and guilt.

In addition, a greater sense of choice allows us to connect more easily with our genuine selves. It is hard to explore our more authentic selves if we are afraid we will find something that might see us punished when we are dead.

Taking this further, without concerns about an afterlife, we can better explore new ideas in philosophy, science and metaphysics. Not believing in an afterlife allows us to free our minds and explore existence virtually unrestrained.

I would now like you to write down the positives of not believing in an afterlife.

Positives
1. ....
2. ....
3. ....
4. ....

Living and then not existing might not be such a bad thing.

b. Our Consciousness Lives On

If you believe there is an afterlife, what are some positives?

We have already considered a few. For instance, the people we love are never gone; they are absent for only a short time.

Accumulating material things doesn't become worth our time; we realise that people matter most since they go on and the material stuff doesn't. There is less status anxiety. We, again, focus more on connection.

The next life can be something to look forward to as a natural part of existence. There is the promise of more to come.

We open ourselves up to more profound spiritual connections and insight. The spirit goes on and has much to notice and experience even beyond the physical realm. This is something we can tap into now too.

We can prepare for life in this realm so that everyone has a more satisfying experience. If we know we come back, why not make it the best it can be for next time? If people are doing it tough, it could be us next time.

We open ourselves up to more love. We don't have to fear losing our love for everyone and everything since, ultimately, they never leave us.

Now write down the positives of believing in an afterlife here.

Positives
1. ....
2. ....
3. ....
4. ....

As we have seen, if the brain only sees the threat of loss, it makes us afraid. However, if the benefits outweigh the losses, the fear dissolves away.

So, whenever you feel afraid of death, think of the positives within the confines of whatever belief you have. Then, perhaps, if you are ready, reconsider your views so that fear of death is no longer a burden you carry.

If we still fear death or are too scared by it to even face it, then we try step 10.

Step 10. Harry Potter It

If death holds too many demons or too much pain, use art to tame it.

As we have seen, art holds enormous potential for self-exploration and expression. It also offers an excellent way to change our story, making us less afraid. Traditionally this has been true, and it can be true again.

Listen to the tales of what happens to us after we die, and we can find many rich and beautiful stories. For instance, some Australian first peoples tell a tale of their relatives travelling into the sky and watching us here below. We see them in the flickering of the stars. Other such tribal beliefs include the passing spirits still walking among us and remaining connected to a part of the Country. That is why they may ask permission of the ancients before walking on their land.

But, some of you may be thinking, the tales from ancient tribes aren't true; they are primitive and naïve.

Can't our modern beliefs about the afterlife also be regarded as primitive and naïve?

Consider what is more important to us in our stories of death. Are they to help us to live the most satisfying life we can, one without unnecessary fear and suffering, or are they told to terrorise people into following a set of rules that often benefit a select few?

If we set the benchmark, the story or beliefs we hold must work for us. They must help us grow and improve as human beings. From that perspective, many traditional cultural beliefs about death can be regarded as some of the most practical and refined in the world. They work.

As our traditional ancestors once did, look into song, stories, painting, sculpture and dance. Express the positive aspects of both life and death and bring them into the physical realm of this world. We can expect many of our fears regarding death to disappear by doing so.

Take your time.

*****

Alan found calling the bluff of death to be most helpful. Like many of us, he'd never looked into the possibilities and let them play out. Now he could see the positives and the negatives. With more insights, he was quickly able to find acceptance. Then, suddenly, he wasn't afraid of stomach upsets anymore. He now goes to restaurants and can visit his family without worrying whether he'll have an attack of debilitating fear.

* * * * *

We live in an age of a pandemic that forces many of us to face our mortality. This can trigger many debilitating fears, including one of the greatest we may know: the fear of death. But the fear of death doesn't have to be a torment. It can be a blessing and an opportunity. Now we finally get to know ourselves and our sense of place in the world better than ever. Facing the fear of death can offer profound, life-changing insights.

What has taming your fear of death taught you?

* * * * *

Now we tackle any remaining fears related to Covid.

CHAPTER 17

NO! NOT COVID!

For Ash Jackson, the arrival of Covid took a terrifying turn. Up until the pandemic Ash, a 48-year-old musician, made a living with music productions, gigs in Melbourne suburbs, playing in cover bands and teaching guitar. Then Melbourne imposed a six-week lockdown. Suddenly, no work. No going out. Lots of time on the internet. She was already a self-professed loner. Ten years previously, the church she belonged to as a born-again Christian ousted her once she came out as transgender. Being even more isolated during the lockdown, she found her community online in the anti-lockdown movement. She was fully into it, regularly being on the frontline at 'freedom' rallies, putting her body on the line. Was she scared? At home, she'd barricade the doors with a couch and tables and booby-trapped the windows. Then an incident at a rally changed her view of the movement entirely.

In May 2021, Ash attended a 'freedom' protest. Other 'freedom' movement members encouraged her to throw herself in front of the police, despite a move-on notice. She did. Then 'they all buggered off and left me'. She felt confused. Because she'd been cooperative, the police let her off. A week later, she was arrested for her role in organising protests and publishing an anti-police booklet online. The police didn't treat her as she expected. They shared with Ash their concerns for their families and the difficulties of working in the frontline in a pandemic. They sympathised with her struggle with her gender and mental health. Police even regularly did welfare checks after she was released. They were not the Gestapo she thought they were. She'd been wrong about them.

Sceptical, she checked online and found out about the substantial amount of money made by people in conspiracy movements. She decided to leave the 'freedom' movement. Suddenly, an enormous weight lifted from her shoulders.

On reflection, she described being part of this conspiracy movement as totally soul-destroying. She lost a lot of friends and fell out with her family; she missed her nieces most. Fortunately, her family was quick to welcome her back.

*****

As we have noted, the fears from Covid can affect each of us in different ways. Petra was terrified to go to school, contract the virus and die, leaving her children without a mother. Brian's social anxiety worsened after working more than a year at home and having minimal face-to-face contact. For Leo, like Ash, anxiety manifested along a conspiratorial line. Covid has triggered or highlighted many fears.

But isn't fear or anxiety related to Covid normal?

Sure, you'd have to be a robot or in cryostasis – frozen like a popsicle – for news of Covid to not have brought at least some worry or concern. After all, our world was turned upside down. Our lives have been riddled with uncertainty. How long would the lockdowns last? Was the virus in my suburb? Were the children safe to go back to school? Would I keep my job and be able to make a living? So, of course, Covid was going to evoke a fear response. The issue, though, is the level of anxiety Covid has triggered. Has it restricted our lives – held us back from living? If it has, then fear related to Covid isn't just an annoyance, an inconvenience or something we can cast aside. It is a significant illness that needs to be addressed, or we continue to suffer needlessly.

In other words, do we want to live with the level of fear Covid has triggered, in whatever form that might be? Do you?

By now, you will have a fair idea of what it means to tame fear. You will have noticed that anxiety is triggered by our brains running through scenarios that predict terrible consequences. Our brain loves to prepare us for its worst cases. And until we give it what it wants, the fear remains.

Thankfully, we have not only learned what fear wants from us, but also developed skills to answer it.

Covid-related fears are no different from other fears; they want the same answers. Unless our fears are particularly extreme, such as those arising from trauma, often the skills we have mastered already will suffice. We will look at how to tackle fears related to PTSD next.

Of course, I'm assuming you still have Covid-related fears.

You may have already resolved some or all of your Covid-related fears by now. You may have done this in the preceding chapters as you learned the 10 steps or tamed them within the mini-workbook pages. You could have already resolved them in the chapter devoted to taming fears related to illness, or in the previous chapter where we tamed our fear of death. If so, good for you. In that case you can consider this chapter to be a revision and an opportunity to refine a few methods.

However, if significant Covid-related fears remain for you, we can now focus on them.

Our approach will be similar to previous chapters; we will work through 10 steps.

10 Steps to Taming Covid-related Fears

Step 1. Find a Safe Place

Let us assume you have found your physically and mentally safe places. As with tackling any fear, we need to know we will not be disturbed and can retreat to a mentally calm place when we need to.

Step 2. Name It to Tame It

There are so many fears surrounding Covid it can be challenging to know where to begin. As we have done in the past, name the most potent fear for you, the one in your face. If one isn't apparent, wait for one to show up then name it. Once again, we must be as accurate as we can.

Below is a shortlist of Covid-related fears you may wish to consider to see whether they resonate.

Fears about Personal and Family Health and Wellbeing

- Fear we or our loved ones will die or get severely ill.
- Fear of another lockdown meaning we will not see our interstate or overseas loved ones for a long time.
- Fear of another lockdown meaning if a loved one falls ill we will not be able to help them or, worse, see them before they die.

- Fear of the vaccines: efficacy, safety, and short-term and long-term side effects.
- Fear of the treatments: efficacy, safety, and short-term and long-term side effects.
- Fear of having no choice – being in an increasingly authoritarian government. We either get vaccinated or have restrictions on what we can do and where we can go.
- Fear of being a guinea pig of the pharmaceutical companies.

Fears about Community and Spread
- Fear of the risk of a new variant emerging.
- Fear of another lockdown and further or renewed restrictions.
- Fear of losing our job or that our career will suffer.
- Social anxiety fears, such as fear of returning to work (like Brian), uni or school or being in public.
- Fear of passing on the virus.
- Fear of moving around in case we contract and spread the virus.
- Fear this will happen again, only worse.
- Fear of passing the virus onto a vulnerable person, and they die.

Covid offers many potential fears to tame.

Has the above list helped you recognise your fear? Write it down.

My fear is
....

If the fear is particularly potent, I recommend drawing it and giving it a name, as we did earlier with other severe fears.

Don't worry if you think you haven't named the fear correctly. As we have seen, if there are more profound fears, they will surface once we explore.

Please see the preceding appropriate chapters if you fear that you or a loved one will fall ill or die.

Step 3. Reality-check the Fairies and Unicorns

Covid has released many fairies and pink unicorns. Our worst-case-prone minds have struggled to make sense of what is happening and feel reassured. What has made it especially difficult to ground us has been the issue of trust.

Have you noticed that many of us no longer trust our governments, scientists, pharmaceutical companies and doctors? Be reassured that they primarily have our wellbeing at heart. We have heard so much about corruption and a focus on profit ahead of people's wellbeing that it has left us sceptical, distrusting and disillusioned. We no longer know who to believe in. Not all countries have these trust issues.

For instance, Denmark has a high level of trust in government and medical expertise. It also has a robust social security system, which is a strong indication that people's welfare matters. As a result, compared with Australians, Danes have greater confidence that their government, health professionals and scientists aren't being controlled by special interests.

By comparison, the USA has one of the worst social security systems in the western world. It blatantly puts profit ahead of individual safety and wellbeing. Unfortunately, in the USA the government and pharmaceutical companies have conducted unethical experiments on their own people, such as the Tuskegee Syphilis Study conducted on African American men by the US Government from 1932 to 1972.

This is certain to erode trust. In addition, the prevalence of pharmaceutical lobbying of government is the highest in the world. How can the people fully trust a government that is clearly being bought by big pharma?

If we can't trust people in authority, we can be expected to look for answers and reassurance elsewhere, such as the internet. We mentioned previously the problem of our fantasy-prone minds going crazy with Dr Google. All too easily, the masses of information we see online can lead to confusion and, worse, entirely unrealistic views, beliefs and interpretations. And with these fantastical ideas come severe levels of fear.

How can we counter these fear-motivated fantasies?

We can begin by reality testing our fear. We can ask, is our fear reasonable?

We can find a health professional we trust, such as our family doctor. Ask them questions. If you know they have your best interests at heart and are well informed, they can help stomp out many fantasies. The earlier you ask your trusted source, the better. We should do this before we are so invested in the unrealistic dream that it is hard to shake.

A consultant I know who works in the approval process for veterinary pharmaceuticals received a call from her good friend. The consultant's job is to find data that pharmaceutical companies want to hide. Her friend called wanting to know about the efficacy of Ivermectin, a worming medication, in the treatment of Covid. They informed the consultant that they had read online that many intelligent people had looked at the data and were sure of Ivermectin's efficacy. Unfortunately, none of the clever people had a medical or research background. The consultant gently reminded her friend that not all the data available online is all of the company's data, including products like Ivermectin. Besides, as it turned out, the data surrounding Ivermectin was falsified. The results were faked. It still hasn't been shown to work against Covid.

Why do so many of us believe in treatments that have been tested and shown not to work? There are several reasons. Chief among them, a story of hope relieves our fear. If there are many easy-to-acquire treatments out there, we have less reason to be afraid. It is more soothing to believe that government and pharma are holding back treatments than to face the unresolved fears of illness and even death.

Remember, our brain doesn't know what is real. Therefore, it will adopt the story that offers it a greater chance of survival even if the story is fantastical.

Thankfully, the friend trusted the consultant's expertise. It soothed her troubled mind.

Consider the following recommendations to help you reality check your Covid-related fear:

- Keep an open mind.
- Search for more information. Search out several fact-checking sites, such as those from the Australian ABC or Australian Associated Press, RMIT Factlab and Agence France-Press (AFP).
- Don't go looking to prove you are right. Instead, try to prove you are wrong; see the other possibilities.
- Be open to the opinions of people with expertise in their field. If you think their views or statements have been tainted by money, then seek out a different knowledgeable and experienced expert – one in whom you have faith.

How did we go? Is your fear still here? If it is, let us consider step 4.

Step 4. Have a Sit-down

Don't forget to sit down with your fear and notice how it makes you feel. Make space for it. Hold it in your presence. Don't let it escape.

Now we can have a chat.

Step 5. Have the Chat and Ask the Primary Question

Let's get straight to the question. You know it by now.

What do you need from me for the fear to go away?

Does an image come to mind, an answer or answers? Remember, the answer must be realistic – achievable. Whole-body transplant and travel to a Covid-free world are out. So are magical powers. Sorry.

Maybe the solution is to visit a trusted specialist, such as your family physician, as mentioned previously. Perhaps it is to stop using the internet as a source of information.

If your fear has a solution, write down what you can do.

To resolve my fear, I can:
1. ....
2. ....
3. ....
4. ....

Put the plan it wants from you into place. Then, commit to it.

Are you ready for acceptance? Are you prepared to say I have tried everything reasonable; there is nothing more I can do? If you have and you genuinely believe it, you will know relief.

If our fear remains, we call its bluff.

Step 6. Call Fear's Bluff

OK, your worst Covid-related fear comes true. What's your plan?

By now, it will be familiar that there are two main ways to call a fear's bluff: a direct approach or an indirect approach.

Direct Approach

Are you ready and willing to let your Covid-related fear give you its worst? Are you ready to not hold back and instead let the ghost of your fear wear itself out inside you? Are you willing to let it emotionally shout at you and fade?

If you are, now is the time. First, follow the steps outlined previously in Chapter 11.

If you aren't ready to be so direct, we try the indirect approach.

Indirect Approach

What is your plan? You know by now that the fear will remain until we give it one.

Don't forget, we still need to access the emotions of the scenario we are afraid of. A critical part of using the indirect approach is the need to feel the fear of the worst case, then ask questions – to step inside the balloon fear monster. We explore to help our brain see other options and perspectives from the inside. We can't do this by being rational and emotionally detached about it.

To help our brain consider its options, here is a small example of questions specific to dealing with Covid-related fears. In addition, you may wish to ask the questions we asked about fears related to illness in Chapter 15.

Some questions we could ask include:

- If I get vaccinated, will my fear of Covid reduce?
- What can I do to allay my fears about the vaccine?
- When I look back on this in five or ten years, will I have a different way of looking at the fear I have now?
- Can I choose to have the vaccine for other reasons besides having to for my work or because the government says so, such as because I see personal benefits for my family and me? Will having the vaccine for those other reasons alleviate my fear?
- If a family member or I get Covid, what is my plan? What will I do?
- What can I reasonably do to prevent getting Covid?
- What plan can I put in place in case of another outbreak or lockdown?
- What strategies will I use for my worsened social anxiety and fear of returning to uni or work?
- If the fear of Covid triggers – brings up – any past fears, what are they, and how do I tame them?

Remember, be inquisitive. Try to help your brain get as complete and realistic a picture as possible about what it is afraid of and the circumstances around it. Rather than rely on unreliable hearsay and false hope, have an honest look at what can and can't be done.

Please avoid denial for the reasons outlined earlier.

Do you have any other questions you might need to ask your fear to help better understand and resolve it?

If so, write them down here.

1. ....
2. ....
3. ....
4. ....

Don't forget, come back to the questions every day until the fear is resolved – tamed. Then, change the questions if new ones come to mind. Find what works. Talk to your fear using your emotional simulator, as mentioned earlier.

There is no shame in seeking trusted help when you feel you need it.

*****

Do you have a plan your fear can agree with? Is your fear significantly less? If so, great.

Perhaps you have exhausted all realistic options – every last one. If you have, then can you finally allow acceptance? Can you see that there is nothing more you can do?

Don't forget, acceptance can't be faked. Our brain has to run through the scenarios in its emotionally connected simulator and see that absolutely no option exists or is worthwhile. If you still feel fear, it means your brain still sees it can do something. It is then up to us to find out what that option is and see whether it truly is realistic. All the steps we have learned so far will help our brains do this.

Persist. This is a challenge, not a pass or fail on an exam.

If calling the bluff of our Covid-related fear has not helped, we try simulator magic.

Step 7. Rehearse Success: Simulator Magic

Are you afraid of needles? I know many who are. It isn't a silly fear. This might be your Covid-related fear: your fear of needles may be preventing you from having the vaccine. But fear of needles is one we can reduce by rehearsing success.

Apply the step we learned to rehearse success earlier.

1. Write down the outcome you are afraid of.

   I am afraid the following will happen
   ....

2. Write down what success looks like.

   Success for me means
   ....

3. Rehearse the physical steps – realistically – of what success looks like, of you succeeding. Then, keep repeating it over and over in your mind.
4. Every time the fear of failure comes up, replace it with the image and feeling of success.

For example, if we fear needles, we may worry about the pain of the needle or passing out, as we might have done before. Success will mean that we know the pain is trivial, fleeting or nothing compared to stubbing our toe. The pain is so tiny we don't notice it or our attention is elsewhere, meaning the needle isn't on our mind. Would you like a lollypop to suck on before you have the needle? Sometimes the sugar helps and is a distraction. Perhaps success looks like having the needle while lying on a bed, so we know we won't pass out. We can imagine success as walking out of the room, having had our needle and getting on with our day. In the scheme of things, the needle wasn't worth thinking about.

Rehearse your success, not your failure, for whatever fear remains for you.

Remember the good wolf versus the bad wolf. First, put your energies on the good wolf, the success, and what it looks and feels like. Then, every time the fear arises, repeatedly focus on the positive image. Don't forget, your thoughts only have the power you give them.

If you have a plan to counter your fear, rehearse your success. Make it the preferred neural pathway for the brain to use when the need arises. That will increase your chance of success.

If rehearsing success isn't helpful, we move on to step 8.

Step 8. Combat Memory Shenanigans

Will desensitisation help you resolve your Covid-related fear?

That will depend on the fear.

If our worry is that a vulnerable family member will get Covid, then there isn't much we can desensitise. However, if the fear is around a location, such as being in a hospital, then desensitisation can help.

Are there any fears related to the illness that you think will benefit from desensitisation? If so, write them here.

1. ....
2. ....
3. ....

Take your time and work on desensitisation yourself, as outlined previously. Don't forget, if you have any problems, you can seek trusted professional help.

Step 9. Create a Joyous New Picture

You know the drill. It is time to use the joy switch.

If we are afraid, we can guarantee that until now we have focused on what will go wrong – all the negatives. But we need to see positives to make our brain simulation realistic.

To help us see some positives, let us consider some of the possible Covid-related fears we named earlier.

FEAR	POSITIVE SCENARIO – JOY SWITCH ON
Fear of suffering long-term side effects from the vaccine or treatment	We will still be alive. Having the vaccine or treatment allowed us a better chance to survive. We can appreciate life.
Fear of a new lockdown	It will give us more time to get to know ourselves and work on reducing our fears. It is an opportunity to reconsider our direction and future.
Fear of losing our job	We have a chance to upskill or find a new career path. We may find a part-time job is better for work-life balance. A new job may mean new friends.
Fear of social anxiety increasing the longer we are away from others	This is a chance to improve our small talk and friendship skills so when we are out there again, we will be better liked.
Fear of passing on the virus to a vulnerable person	We can become more careful about hygiene and self-care. We can learn to do all that is reasonable to prevent us from spreading the virus so we can accept we have done enough.
Fear this will happen again, only worse	This gives us a new challenge to help us grow and develop increasing insight and understanding about ourselves as a human being. We use the opportunity to connect more with ourselves, others and nature. We learn our priorities and reshape them if needed.

I know a young carpenter who was a chronic Mr Negative. Every week he'd talk about how things weren't as they used to be or he wanted them to be. Not surprisingly, he suffered depression. It was so bad his parents were convinced he'd not survive. Then we made an agreement. Every week he would write a list of all the positives of his week, including what he did OK or better than expected. It could be going out and socialising even if he didn't feel like it. It could be going to a work site run by his mates even though he thought he couldn't contribute. No complaining allowed. No focus on the negatives. He was to focus on positives and solutions, rather than be drawn into the negativity of the problem and dwell there.

After severe depression for years, he was significantly better within two weeks. Then, within two months, he was back to his old self, only wiser for the counselling and insights gained over the years. He now reminds his friends, don't tell me the problems, tell me the solutions. Turning on the joy switch and focusing on the positives has power that transforms beyond taming fear.

If we are struggling to turn on the joy switch, maybe we need to look at who we are communicating with.

Are we online and only chatting to, or getting information from, doom merchants? Or do we connect only with those focusing on the negatives of life and some impending apocalypse? If so, we should reconsider our friends and information sources. Hang out with the negative, and it rubs off. On the other hand, hang out with those who are more realistic and upbeat, and we can be the same; take the positive vibes from them.

Mind you, I don't think many positive and reasonable people are going to want to hang around a Mr or Ms Glum. So perhaps we should make sure our joy switch has had some practice first.

Remember, every fear can be reframed and seen in a positive light. The more the brain sees what it gains, the less it has to fear, and our fear resolves.

If you are still struggling to turn your joy switch on because of fear, seek a health professional to help.

Suppose all the above steps haven't been as beneficial as we hoped. Maybe we are so scared by our fear we can barely face it. Then we use the healing powers and potential of art.

Step 10. Harry Potter It

If the fear is hard to face or budge, as we have seen we can always change it with art and creativity.

Decide what artform you want to use to explore the nature of what you feel and let it out. Maybe it will be storytelling, painting, poetry, sculpture, music or dance, or any combination of any forms of expression.

Once again, don't express yourself to an audience. Instead, this is you connecting with your deeper self and bringing it into the conscious world.

If it is a fictional story, don't forget to show what the main characters had to experience or understand in order to transform. Similarly, if it is a painting or drawing, express the curing process as much as the fear, sorrow, terror or other feelings.

Pick a feeling or perspective you want to go into and set aside a week or more to devote to it until you feel it has been released. Some people I know write or otherwise express themselves one day per week. Make room for whatever feelings come up so you can hold them.

As mentioned earlier, there are professional art and music therapists to help. If you get stuck or need to do this with others you can trust, then give them a call.

* * * * *

The secrets and insights into the fundamentals of fear have been invaluable. They have helped Ellie tame her everyday fear of never seeing her children again once they exit the door, helped Kallie tame her fear of regret, assisted Max in compartmentalising and gave Stan an off-switch for his busy mind. They have offered Brian a way to overcome social anxiety worsened after months of isolation. They also helped us to see how connecting with nature calms us, as it did for Mandy from Canada, Josh overworked in IT, and Jess on her personal journey. Melinda who was trapped in the depths of despair from uncontrolled anxiety found relief and reclaimed her life. Roberto just needed to answer two questions to stop fear bothering him. And Bec could visit a doctor with more confidence once her fear was resolved. The secret insights were especially powerful for Ken, allowing him to overcome his fear of illness. They helped guide Alan and allowed him to peer inside his anxiety and master his fear of death.

Finally, the skills we gained have helped us overcome our fears in a challenging time: the age of Covid. A modern pandemic has given us an opportunity to understand and master methods that go beyond calming fears or acting despite them. It has given us the ability to resolve fears – to resolve and erase them so they never again significantly impact our lives. It has liberated us from a cage of our mind's making.

Although all these achievements are worthy, this is not the final chapter. There is a side of fear we haven't explored yet that is more severe than many of us may ever have to face. It is the fear associated with severe trauma, such as those that trigger the severely debilitating condition known as PTSD.

CHAPTER 18

I ONLY JUST SURVIVED! TAMING THE FEAR OF SEVERE TRAUMA AND PTSD

Norbert – a tall, lean, fit fellow with a pronounced Germanic accent – had been troubled by anxiety for at least six years. He had regular nightmares, was often agitated and avoided anything that reminded him of sick people. In fact, Norbert had now become almost obsessed with his health and was terrified of having something seriously wrong with him. He wasn't always like this; most of his life he had been carefree, calm, well prepared and excited to try new things. That was until his best friend had a heart attack while cycling with him, and Norbert had to do CPR. Although he saved his friend's life, since that day even the mere thought of that moment brought a sense of dread and terror he couldn't control. He'd tried medications and some therapy, but nothing helped. Norbert was being tormented by one of the most insidious and difficult to control fears of all. You may know it as PTSD.

*****

PTSD, post-traumatic stress disorder, is a particularly nasty and powerful fear disorder that can be notoriously hard to cure. Perhaps you are familiar with it being a condition suffered by combat veterans who have had an experience so personally traumatic their minds won't let it go. But anyone can suffer PTSD.

If we experience a significant threat to our lives or safety, PTSD can result.

Many traumas can trigger PTSD, from childhood abuse to sexual assault. It could be from witnessing something traumatic or being in a terrible motor vehicle accident. For Norbert, the trigger was his friend having a heart attack and being the only one there to save his life. Doing CPR on his friend brought home to him his own mortality, that he might die at any moment. It was a fear he couldn't shake.

It should be pointed out that a trauma will not always lead to PTSD. Our brain can resolve many fears triggered by trauma. Much of the time, we can overcome the trauma within weeks without serious effects. However, when the fears persist for at least a month without respite, we may need to consider whether we have PTSD.

PTSD, like other mental illnesses, is diagnosed based on symptoms. There are no physical tests, such as blood tests or brain imaging scans, to say we suffer it.

What are some of the typical symptoms of PTSD?

Typical symptoms include re-experiencing the event, known as flashbacks. Those who suffer it will say it is like we are there again. We have recurring dreams about the event. We avoid places, occurrences or people to avoid distressing memories, feelings or thoughts about the original event.

Further, we become so on edge that we can easily become aggressive and detach from those close to us. Finally, we become reckless or self-destructive, such as taking extreme risks or abusing alcohol or drugs.

Unfortunately, we can blame others for our situation or be overly critical of ourselves. We can also withdraw and shut down, not wanting to do anything.

PTSD is a horrible illness. It is horrid for the sufferer as well as those close to them, who can struggle to support them.

Why devote a separate chapter to PTSD?

First, because PTSD and the fear it elicits are so extreme, but also because it can be challenging to navigate out of.

The aim here is not to offer a comprehensive way out of PTSD or other severe trauma-related conditions; that would be beyond a book of this nature. Instead, consider this chapter as a supplement, especially if you feel stuck.

This is where the secrets we learned earlier about fear become invaluable.

Yes, understanding the fight or flight response helps PTSD make perfect sense. Our brain is still in the mode of running away or taking the person down. But that insight doesn't necessarily offer a road map to recovery. Simply trying to lessen the fear response isn't going to fix the problem, nor will medication. Yes, there are other treatment approaches, and we'll consider them in a moment. But understanding fear in ways considered at the beginning of the book can likely offer us a greater depth of insight and direction perhaps not otherwise considered and can further guide our recovery.

Let us break down how to tame severe trauma, and PTSD fear, into two parts:

1. Demystifying the Ugly: I've Blown the Fuse Box
2. Using a Map: Want a Compass Anyone?

The first part will use our new insights about fear to help make sense of what happens in severe trauma and PTSD. The second part is how we can put these insights to practical use.

1. Demystifying the Ugly: I've Blown the Fusebox

Oh, no. Too many Christmas lights. I've blown the fuse box!

Overload our brain, and it's designed to switch off – not literally, but close.

How does our brain respond to severe trauma? What can we expect?

The first thing to learn about our brain's reaction to trauma, or our response manifesting as PTSD, is that it is a normal, expected response. There is nothing mysterious about it.

According to the secrets we learned earlier, our brain is made to react to fear in predictable ways.

What happens when we are severely traumatised, such as when we almost die in a car crash, we have bullets whizz past our head, bombs explode near us or a knife is put to our throat? First, our brain says I need to survive this NOW.

Then it says I need to prevent this happening again, or I'll be toast.

In other words, during the event we have a massive adrenalin rush; we are faster and stronger and can think more clearly – at least initially. We get out of there if we can. We take shelter if needed. If we are able to, we fight back as trained and we defend ourselves and our mates. We do what we need to do, and we are hyped up to the max to make it happen.

Aggression and anger are feelings we can tap into when we fight for our lives to see us through.

Being petrified, shaking and unable to move can prevent us from doing something dangerous and make matters worse.

Then, we survive. The threat has passed.

But not in our mind.

It has a new memory of the future of the worst kind. It has one or more prediction scenarios that look abysmal. It is desperate to find answers. This event might happen again at any moment.

WHERE'S MY PLAN?
WHERE'S MY PLAN?
WHERE'S MY PLAN?

Cue our fear monster of the most potent type.

Explaining the Symptoms

What Is a Flashback?

A flashback is a reactivation of pathways in our brain that were laid down during a terrifying event or circumstance. It is a memory activated with the emotion attached. Of course, it feels like we are there again; that is how memories work. The fear is extreme this time because so is/was the threat. The brain makes sure it remembers what almost ended us. It is quick to bring it again to the surface. We don't forget.

Any event, place, person, picture, film, object or smell that is similar to what we noticed during the original trauma can trigger a flashback.

Why Do We Have Recurring Dreams of the Event?

As we learned earlier, our brain is trying to find its way out. It is trying to find a solution. To do that, it needs to reactivate the memory and explore alternatives. Solutions will likely feel extreme since the event and feelings were extreme. We may know the brain as it explores these alternatives as suffering nightmares. The nightmares continue until the brain has what it needs.

Why Do We Avoid Some Places and Events?

Our brain reactivates memories according to people and events around us, to circumstance. If, for instance, the trauma involved seeing a young child being seriously hurt in an accident, then seeing a young child of a similar age will reactivate the memory and bring up associated thoughts and feelings. If these thoughts and feelings disturb us, we will avoid seeing, or being around, children of that age or appearance.

Not all avoidance will have an associated flashback. We may only notice the discomfort as our brain relives the scenario in our subconscious. We simply avoid what makes us feel uncomfortable, whether or not we are aware of its cause.

Why Do We Emotionally Detach?

We emotionally detach because we blew the fuse box.

We can't live if we are so scared that we can't move, sleep or eat. If we constantly live in terror and are paralysed, we will die.

To survive, the brain shuts down what emotions and feelings it can. It means that, metaphorically, while the refrigerator and a few lights can stay on, the fuses to the stereo, TV, computer, iron, washing machine and drier will be blown.

Fear from severe trauma overloads our brain and makes it go into a partial shutdown, just as your computer can go into safe mode after it freezes. We can access a few essential functions in safe mode, but we can't use higher-end programs, such as complex video and graphics. Sorry, no video games. The same applies to our brain experiencing emotional detachment.

The side effect of the partial shutdown is that we feel life as distant and vague, and we aren't all there. It is like being an observer, on the outside. We notice it happening, but it appears to be happening to someone else.

The problem is if we stay detached, life can be a misery – not just for us but those around us too.

Ken, who we mentioned earlier, had a fear of severe illness. As a result, he would at times feel detached, which increased his fear. Once his fear was resolved, the detachment left.

Why the Aggression and the Anger?

Aggression and anger can keep us alive. For example, a soldier in combat can use anger and aggression to keep them motivated and fight off the enemy. Anger, when focused, is fear funnelled to give us greater strength, speed, reaction time, awareness and presence.

Anger and aggression can also be linked to fear. For instance, if we feel fear, it can automatically trigger aggression and anger at any level. Why? Because aggression and anger are what feeling fear was associated with in the past, when we needed fear most just to survive. The more we associate the feeling of fear with aggression and anger, the more likely we will become aggressive and angry when we feel fear. It becomes our brain's automatic response to feeling anxiety, like the way we are trained to automatically stop when we are approaching a red light while driving.

This is why a soldier who is used to surviving on anger and aggression can get angry and aggressive at not being able to pay the bills or when cut off unexpectedly on the road by another driver. Any fear trigger can become an anger and aggression trigger. As you can imagine, this aggressive response might work well in combat, but it won't go down well at home or in regular life. Soon it can make people afraid to be near us, and we end up alone.

Why the Reckless Self-abuse?

There are many reasons for reckless self-abuse. For example, we may want to punish ourselves for what we have done. Many of us come from families or communities where we expect punishment. If we don't get it, we feel uncomfortable. So, we punish ourselves, or we may want to escape.

Abusing alcohol, as we noted earlier, is used as a common method of escape from anxiety, as are other types of drugs and adrenalin-triggering activities. When we struggle to deal with niggling fear and impending terror every moment of the day, we may seek out another fear to drown out the one bothering us. Besides, the new adrenalin rush will make us feel alive and present again if we are detached. It can wake us up. It can also become addictive.

Adrenalin is one of the most addictive substances known to man. More addictive than heroin or smoking. They don't call the people who jump off cliffs with parachutes or climb flat rock faces without ropes adrenalin junkies for nothing.

Being reckless can also be because we don't care anymore; we don't worry about the consequences. We don't consider them anyway because we are detached, or they aren't as important as the need for the rush. Unfortunately, reckless behaviour can take our life. And our friends and family will struggle to understand and support actions they know won't end well.

Why the Quickness to Blame Others?

PTSD sufferers may be quick to blame others. If the problem isn't our fault, we don't need to change. If we don't need to change, we don't need to face our problems.

Blaming others means we don't need to face the fear monster again and be traumatised by it over and over. So, if it is someone else's problem, at least we don't have to face the fear.

Coping Strategies

Norbert was suffering many of the symptoms of severe trauma. He had nightmares, agitation, flashbacks and avoidance. His brain just couldn't find what it needed, and he was suffering because of it. Thankfully, his fear didn't manifest as aggression, blame or reckless behaviours.

As we've noted, these symptoms are normal. They are normal in that they are what we might expect our brain to do in reaction to fear that is so severe and scenarios so terrible that our brain can't get rid of them. We call them coping mechanisms or strategies. This is our brain trying to cope and get by, trying to keep us alive and be safe.

Unfortunately, our coping strategies don't often help us get the most out of life. They don't always work for us. For instance, smashing walls out of anger or aggression isn't an excellent way to deal with our partner moving in with their parents for a few weeks, nor is blaming them or anyone else we can find, or closing us away from everyone who cares.

Of course, once the fear has been resolved, our brain no longer needs to use the unhelpful coping strategies that make life such misery.

Complex PTSD and Trauma

By now, you may think resolving PTSD or trauma is simply about overcoming the fear triggered by the horrible event, like Norbert overcoming the fear triggered by his friend almost dying in front of him. If we were well previously, and a single event triggered our ongoing fear, then taming that one fear makes all the difference. But, for many of us, there can be more than one fear-triggering incident. Sometimes there can be a lifetime of them. In that case, we have our work cut out for us. When there are many fears from many traumatic events, we call it complex trauma or complex PTSD. This is a different, and more resistant and troublesome monster altogether.

If the fear from one trauma can trap us in a cage, the fears from many traumas chain us in a locked fortress where someone buried the key.

By the time I met Liza – in her late fifties – she'd been abandoned or rejected by every therapist and mental health service she had approached, even the psychiatric unit at our local hospital. Every day for more than three years, she threatened to kill herself. Not a day went by when she didn't say she couldn't cope anymore. She hated herself with a passion.

Every moment of each day for Liza was unpredictable. She'd either curl up on her bed sobbing or be so agitated she'd walk the streets, often in her pyjamas. Frequently, she would be so distressed she would dissociate and not move all day. Her history was tragic.

Sexual, physical and emotional abuse began at a young age and persisted into her teens. Once she reached puberty, to find love Liza would have sex with anyone who obliged. Only later did she realise she was being used; sex does not equal love. She abused alcohol to quell the emotional torment. She joined the armed services hoping it might settle her. Instead, it made her self-abusive behaviours worse.

For a time, medications worked. The various antidepressants quelled some of the sadness and anxiety enough for Liza to have a semblance of a life. Unfortunately, while the drugs took the edge off, she didn't face her demons. The fears from her trauma were always just beneath the surface. Often we can develop a tolerance to medications, meaning after a while they don't work, and every drug has an upper dose limit.

Several years before I met her, Liza had tried all the medications on the market. One she'd been on for at least five years. Liza said it changed her. When she finally stopped it, she said she couldn't recognise herself in the mirror; it wasn't her. The person she saw was everything she hated, physically and otherwise. And beneath that new face was a person still driven by past terrors.

While the medications were still helping, she married and had a child. Until then, relationships were unstable at best. She loved the father of her child. And she loved her daughter – and still does. Her daughter is now in her twenties. Liza blames herself for her daughter's father hanging himself. She says she must have driven him to it; even though it sounded like he too had his demons and wasn't one to seek help.

What made proper treatment for Liza particularly difficult was being given the label of having a borderline personality disorder (BPD).

What is BPD, and why is it a troublesome diagnosis?

According to DSM-V, a diagnostic manual of mental illness, to have BPD a person needs to have at least five of the following:

- a frantic effort to avoid abandonment, real or imagined
- a pattern of unstable and intense interpersonal relationships

- markedly and persistently unstable self-image or sense of self
- impulsivity, such as unsafe sex and substance abuse
- recurrent suicidal behaviour, gestures or threats
- unstable and markedly reactive mood, such as anxiety, periods of dysphoria (unease and dissatisfaction with life), and irritability lasting a few hours and only rarely a few days
- chronic feelings of emptiness
- difficulty controlling anger
- severe dissociative symptoms.

Liza certainly fits the criterion. The problem with a BPD diagnosis is that once a doctor sees that diagnosis, it can set off alarm bells. It says this person has a chronic condition we cannot cure. So, often, people with BPD are regarded as too challenging to have as patients and too difficult to treat. Patients diagnosed with BPD have told me once the doctor reads the diagnosis in their file, the doctor stops listening to them.

Only in the last few years has it finally been recognised that the reason a person has BPD symptoms is because of complex trauma.

Every symptom in BPD is a coping strategy that doesn't ultimately work. Instead of bringing love, acceptance, care and support, it often creates the opposite: anger, anxiety, uncertainty, loneliness and trying to cope with fear so strong that most of us would struggle to imagine it. This was what Liza experienced.

Complex trauma is fear that is out of control on many fronts. Each fear is difficult to engage with and soothe, let alone resolve.

Complex PTSD is commonly associated with chronic childhood trauma and chronic domestic violence. Liza had known both.

Why do I bring up the diagnosis of complex trauma or complex PTSD?

For several reasons.

First, to remind us that trauma writes on the tablet of who we are. This is especially true in our younger years.

As we have seen, unresolved fears remain. They are associated with scenarios, dreams and images of what will happen next in our future. These are part of the stories we define ourselves by.

For instance, if our parents emotionally neglect us, ignore us or abandon us, our brain is terrified it will happen again. So, like all fears, it searches for a reason why. If it can understand why then it can predict when it might happen again and what it needs to do to prevent it, if it can. But because a child only sees the world from a limited view – and because they have no idea of adult problems – the story our brain creates is that the problem must be us: we are unlovable; we are defective; we will always be abandoned by those we love. Liza's traumatic upbringing caused her to feel this way.

Since this negative story about us is founded on trying to quell fear, the story will remain until the fear is rewritten – resolved. No matter how many people may show they love us, if we have not rewritten that fear, we will have doubts about any love or relationship. We will always expect to be left alone. We may often make it a reality; we rehearse our failure.

Everything we do to a child writes their self-stories, how they see and treat themselves, for a lifetime. Why this is important will become apparent in a moment.

Another reason to raise the diagnosis of complex trauma and PTSD is to remind us not to judge. Instead, to be understanding and compassionate.

To label someone as having BPD is not helpful. What is helpful is to recognise they have multiple levels of fear tormenting them, to see that they are struggling every day to cope and have a regular, satisfying life.

This isn't about sympathy, either. I don't know many sufferers of mental illness who crave sympathy – an 'oh, poor you' response. Punishing the sufferer for their antisocial or inappropriate behaviours is not a helpful strategy either.

We all do it: you hurt me so I'll hurt you back, so you don't do it again. It is an instinct. It forms the foundation of what we know as justice or revenge. But to a person already unjustly punished by abuse, as Liza has been, being punished becomes another trauma.

By the way, not listening to someone – ignoring them or dismissing their suffering – is a form of abuse.

Finally, I bring up the diagnosis of complex PTSD and trauma to remind us that we now have a better understanding of what trauma is and what it does to us. This gives us hope. Yes, fears can trap us and restrict our lives, but once we know what our brain wants, we can help liberate it.

Let us consider some treatment options for complex trauma and PTSD and how the secrets of fear we learned earlier can help guide us.

Using a Map: Want a Compass Anyone?

Norbert agreed to a session of EMDR (eye movement desensitisation and reprocessing). EMDR was established in 1987 as a therapy by psychologist Francine Shapiro after noticing her eye movements while walking in a park decreased the negative emotions of distressing memories. I have been trained in EMDR. It is one of a few proven therapies to treat PTSD. More about that in a moment. Norbert was amazed by the results of EMDR: after just one session, his fear regarding the CPR incident had gone. Even years later, it had never returned. He was eternally grateful.

Treatments for complex PTSD or complex trauma include the following therapies:

- CBT (cognitive behavioural therapy). Essentially CBT changes our thoughts and actions, much like we have been doing throughout this book. Many CBT practitioners follow strict recipes or approaches.
- EMDR. As mentioned above.
- Psychodynamic therapy. Essentially this is a talking therapy where therapists help people gain insight into their lives and present-day problems. They often focus on emotions, thoughts, beliefs and early life experiences.
- Somatic therapy. This is a form of body-centred therapy. It looks at the connection between mind and body and uses both psychotherapy and physical therapies as part of a holistic approach.
- Medications (such as antidepressants or antipsychotics) to calm the level of distress.

In addition, Socratic group therapy is beneficial with complex trauma manifesting as traits of BPD. It is suitable as long as the person is well enough to go to a group session – unlike Liza – and not too socially anxious to be among a group.

The Socratic method involves asking a series of probing questions to identify thoughts and beliefs. It also helps assess the consequences of particular thoughts or behaviours. For instance, if I think everyone is a weak a**hole, not worthy of being around, and abuse them, can I expect to feel lonely? Of course.

These are all worthy therapies. But, as you have gathered, my bias is more towards the talking therapies. I consider medications a last resort.

What added benefit do the insights gained about the secrets of fear offer in treating PTSD and complex trauma?

It offers a road map and compass.

Added Benefits of Fear Secrets

Let us see how our new insights and skills can benefit PTSD and complex trauma.

PTSD

One of the most critical questions when trying to get over PTSD is what are we trying to achieve?

That's easy: to get rid of PTSD.

But what does that mean?

Does ridding ourselves of PTSD mean reducing the symptoms, such as anger, aggression, emotional detachment, mood swings and reckless self-abuse? That can be a monumental task if we don't treat the cause – what drives these symptoms in the first place. Reducing each symptom can take a long time and often it can seem like we aren't getting anywhere. It can be a recipe for hopelessness and frustration. We treat one symptom, and the others are either still there or worse. It is hard to snuff out a fire if the fuel and spark are still there.

This is where our understanding of the secret of fear is invaluable. It helps remind us about the cause of all the symptoms. Treat the cause, and the others are much easier to manage and eliminate. If we don't treat the reason, we can expect the symptoms to come back or remain battling inside us. They will remain under the surface, ready to explode or to burn us at any moment. Knowing how fear works offers PTSD sufferers a destination and how to get there.

What is the destination?

The fear driving the PTSD – trauma – is resolved.

How do we get there?

We use many skills and insights we have already learned and tweak them.

By now you will be familiar with the 10 steps to resolving a fear. We won't repeat them all here in workbook fashion. Instead, we will focus on how to get the most from the steps in resolving the fear from the trauma.

Points of Focus
Step 1. Find a Safe Place

The first step – finding a physical and mentally safe place – is essential. Why? Because we may be so physically distressed, we cannot face any troubling emotions, let alone fear.

Physical trauma leaves a physical memory. The trembling, the agitation, the knot in the stomach is physical. We will struggle to face our fear if the physical symptoms overwhelm us every time we even contemplate looking at our fear. That is why many therapists specialising in trauma will often teach self-soothing techniques before engaging the fear behind the trauma.

For instance, we can use self-tapping. Try it. Give yourself a hug, and then tap your hands on your arms or back at a constant rate and rhythm. The brain finds regular, rhythmical movement with mild stimulation as soothing, just like a baby does.

No, we are not weak if we use self-soothing techniques. On the contrary, we are knowledgeable and practical.

You must feel safe here and now to resolve fear. Make sure you do.

Step 2. Name It to Tame It

Just realising the trauma created the fear is enough for now. What the fear actually represents will come later.

Step 3. Reality-check the Fairies and Unicorns

You can bypass the reality-check step. If a trauma happened, it happened. It was real. The scenarios your brain is worried will happen again are real; they happened in the real world. Remember, the brain does not know time. It assumes that at any moment what happened in the past can happen again, even the events of childhood although we are now an adult.

Step 4. Have a Sit-down

If you aren't ready for the sit-down step, then bypass it. Focus on the self-soothing aspects first. Trauma-related fears are often the most potent of all. As mentioned, to even contemplate them can be intolerable. But, on the other hand, you have already made significant progress if you can sit with your fear.

Let us be realistic. For some of us, being able to sit down with our fear could take weeks, months or longer.

Self-soothing, meditation and mindfulness can be helpful. Yes, those strategies are symptom control not a cure in themselves. They have a longer-term purpose; eventually we want to be able to sit in our fear's presence and engage with it, to chat.

Step 5. Have the Chat and Ask the Primary Question

Put the question out there: what do you need from me for the fear to go away?

Typically, it will want us to be safe. Wonderful. What does being safe look like? How can we make it happen? For example, if we have been physically assaulted, does feeling safe mean learning self-defence classes? If we were in a motor vehicle accident, does it mean doing an advanced driver training course? If we were in combat, does it mean learning to compartmentalise combat mode from living in a peaceful society? Does it mean learning to focus more on the present, realising this is a safe place, and letting our minds recognise that to be true? Does it mean having trusted mates nearby, or that we can call at a moment's notice?

Perhaps the solution is understanding what happened in greater detail. Why did the other person focus on me there and then? What could make someone do this to someone else? Could I spot someone like them again? What didn't I see that led me to be so vulnerable? Why did I go into combat? What was I trying to achieve? Would I do it again? How could I limit the risks more than I did?

Self-harm is not an acceptable solution.

If you have a practical answer, then you have made significant progress.

Step 6. Call Fear's Bluff

Either you are ready to enact this step or you are not. If you aren't, bypass it and move to the next steps. There is no shame in bypassing the step where we call fear's bluff. It is not a sign of weakness in any way.

Calling fear's bluff can give us the space to observe and rewrite the fear simultaneously.

Consider different points of view. What would the perpetrator have to have gone through to act as they did? How could I protect myself if it happened again? What more could I do in a similar situation to feel safe? The more points of view we see, the more realistic and familiar the simulation. Thus, the less the fear.

If we become students of our fear, ready to learn what it can teach us, we automatically learn to master it. We understand what it does and why. We begin to predict what sets off the fear and what relieves it. Studying anxiety as a uni subject isn't necessarily as beneficial as it can make us too detached. As we now recognise, knowing scientifically that fear is a fight or flight response doesn't help us rewrite it.

Another approach is being a comforting adult to our inner child. If our traumatic fears are from childhood, it can be helpful to imagine meeting that scared child as an adult. What would we do for them? How would we soothe them? As they experience the event of their trauma, we can be the caring adult that soothes and comforts them. Imagine it. Feel it. This can be a powerful way to rewrite a traumatic memory of childhood.

Step 7. Rehearse Success: Simulator Magic
If simulating the trauma brings on the fear, what realistic simulation lessens it? In other words, what alternative outcome can we realistically visualise that wouldn't trigger such a fear reaction?

For example, if we imagine kicking an assailant in the nuts, would that lessen the fear of another assault? Would we lessen our chance of someone running up our rear if we gradually slowed down our car rather than braking suddenly, or pressed the brake pedal a few times once stopped to flash the brake light or checked our rear mirror more? Which would be an effective image of successfully avoiding a recurrence of the traumatic event?

If you can imagine a visualisation that nullifies the fears of your trauma, use it. Then practise it repeatedly to replace the image of your potential future failure with the new image of success.

Step 8. Combat Memory Shenanigans
Combatting memory shenanigans can be our most valuable step.

Why can it be so critical?

It can be done in a way that doesn't mean we have to share or describe our trauma experience with our therapist. Instead, it can help us desensitise without having to relive it over and over again from therapy session to therapy session.

The method that helps us make such rapid progress was introduced earlier and helped Norbert: EMDR.

EMDR is so valuable because it desensitises our brain to trauma memory. It also helps us rewrite the story we told ourselves when the trauma happened.

For instance, if our car has been hit from behind many times and it wasn't our fault, we can start to believe we are a terrible driver. That is our story: I am a terrible driver. Every time we stop at lights, or a stop sign, our brain will access the memory of the future that someone will hit us. It will also access the story. It isn't just about stopping feeling afraid. While the story remains, so does the scenario and the fear. EMDR eliminates both.

How does EMDR achieve all this?

Ultimately, we don't know. There is only speculation. However, we know our distress reduces rapidly if we can access our fear and notice the story that goes with it – if we can hold onto the feeling of fear and the story – as we follow the therapist's finger moving irregularly in front of us.

Using EMDR, within an hour, our brain can have a new association: the memory of the trauma and feeling calm. Soon the memory will be difficult to access. The fear is resolved.

EMDR doesn't happen in a first session. It takes time to prepare. If one of your coping strategies is to emotionally detach, then EMDR is less likely to work. If you are physically too distressed to even imagine the fear, then first you may need to use self-soothing or other steps mentioned earlier.

Just to clarify for those who may not know much about EMDR: one thing it is NOT is hypnosis. Hypnosis is a very different therapy technique.

If you suffer from PTSD, consider seeing a trained EMDR therapist. EMDR can settle in weeks what might take years to resolve using other methods.

Graduated desensitisation can help, too, especially in places where we feel afraid. But being calm in areas such as shopping centres, in crowds and in a car won't necessarily be as successful as desensitising to the original fear-invoking event.

Speak to a trained trauma therapist if you can.

Step 9. Create a Joyous New Picture

What are some of the positives of you having your fear? What are the negatives?

Don't just focus on how this fear is interrupting your life. Instead, consider what you can gain from it. Turn on your joy switch as much as your trauma-related fear allows. For example, how will mastering PTSD help you to be better able to face and resolve other fears?

What has the trauma taught you about your priorities: who and what matters most to you? Perhaps it has reminded you how critical it is to have trusted mates to call on – how essential close friendships are.

Significant trauma can make us question our worldview. It can make us re-evaluate everything. This isn't a bad thing; it is an opportunity.

Perhaps our trauma has taught us life is fleeting and worth appreciating more, as it did for Gerard.

Maybe combat has taught us how small and insignificant we are? Perhaps that governments are stupid? Perhaps we need to reconsider what we put our life on the line for?

Changing our worldview is often a terrifying experience. Our worldview makes sense of the world and makes it predictable. Take away our worldview, and the world becomes unpredictable until we develop a new and more practical set of beliefs and views. Until our new view is established, we live in fear of the unknown. Unfortunately, we can expect our brain not to give up its beliefs and stories about the world and us very readily.

Yet, we can often tame our fear best by changing our view – our stories – as we have seen.

Do you need to reconcile the stories you live by so you can feel more accepting and less scared of life, as we did when we reconsidered our views on illness and death?

PTSD may demand we reconsider who we are and our place among all things. What an awesome prospect.

Step 10. Harry Potter It

Sometimes we need baby steps to tackle a severe trauma-related fear. We might not be ready to face it directly, but we can explore the edges to get used to it. For example, we can explore it in art.

As we have noted, expressing our feelings in a physical form means we need to access the feelings to do it. These feelings include fear. In the process of repeatedly accessing the feeling and holding it, we are also getting used to it – desensitising ourselves.

I know of old war veterans who have found it invaluable to paint their concerns and the images troubling them.

You determine how you want to use art to rewrite your fear. Don't forget that there are professionals who can help.

*****

Understanding the secrets of fear offers us greater insight into how to tame PTSD-related fear. It reminds us that we still need to face our fears if we are to resolve them. It provides us many alternative ways to do this. It also reminds us that, ultimately, we are trying to change our brain's stories. At the heart of trauma-related fears are negative stories that need to be rewritten. We are offered a map to see where we are going and why. Finally, we are given a compass to help show us the direction in which to take practical steps.

No matter what method we use to treat PTSD, the PTSD will continue to bother us unless our fears are resolved.

It is similar when dealing with complex trauma.

Complex Trauma

What is the best way to treat complex trauma?

Prevent it. What is the point of giving people life vests after they've already been thrown into rapids miles upstream? Why throw them in the white water in the first place?

As we saw in the example of Liza a moment ago, trauma writes inside us the stories we live by. Her traumas taught her she was a person to hate and was unlovable. Her level of distress made it challenging to access any of her traumatic experiences and rewrite them. All her traumas have made her anxious. All the anxieties have combined and are readily triggered. Until she settles even a tiny bit, she won't be able to resolve any of them.

It is challenging to resolve fears in complex trauma with so many fears combined. One fear can trigger another and another. It is like many small waves combining to create a mega wave able to sink the most giant ships.

Self-soothing in treating complex trauma is essential.

Supporting those with complex trauma in their journey using understanding and empathy is critical. Labels such as BPD should be avoided.

Art therapy may be the only foot in the door.

Having many therapists and allied health professionals to support each other in treating these people is ideal.

Little by little, we can make progress.

Can we completely change these people and eliminate all their distress?

No, and it is unrealistic to imagine we can.

It is well recognised that the first five years of life define most of our personality – who we are. These events lay the foundations we build the rest of our life upon – the stories we live by. We may change some of it, but we can't change it all.

Liza continues to be distressed with her symptoms. Her self-hatred has become a barrier to her progress. When she makes some improvement, she stops doing what has helped her. She admits she doesn't believe she deserves to be well. She hates herself and punishes herself for being weak and doing all the foolish things. Being on a pension, she can't afford to be admitted to a private clinic to explore alternative therapies, such as retrying medications. Her worry with new drugs is they will make her suicidality worse – a realistic fear.

What stops her from ending it all?

She couldn't do it to her daughter.

However, Liza and all those caring for her recognise that maybe she can't be saved. And that is OK.

Complex trauma can leave us in such a bottomless pit that not all of us can climb out. There can be too much fear and self-defeating stories to obstruct our recovery.

That is why prevention must be our primary focus in treating complex PTSD. Unfortunately, once all the fears have accumulated, there may be too much damage to fix, as with Liza.

What kind of preventative measures might we focus on? Here are a few suggestions I'm sure many of you have considered:

- Provide increased parental support and education. Help parents rather than blame them. We all need to work to prevent childhood traumas.
- Prioritise a close and supportive community. If there is more love and care, there will be less violence and trauma.
- Provide more funding and training placements to already overwhelmed mental health services. There is so much preventable mental illness, but our services are already overwhelmed.

- Provide a basic income to fall back upon that is above poverty levels. It is well documented that mental illness levels reduce if there is less financial stress.

Too many, like Liza, will need intense mental health support unless we focus on prevention.

In the meantime, we can only master and tame each fear as best we can.

CHAPTER 19

CHOICE AND HOPE

The red dirt road was narrow and about a car and a half in width. It was bordered on each side by dried, crispy grass that crunched under foot and, beyond the grass, by fence lines. My job was to walk among the knee-high grass and the branches, and past old trees to move cattle at least twenty times bigger than me. I'd shout and wave my arms. The cows would dump shit as they ran or tried to avoid me. Some would gush pee. We wouldn't push them too hard, or they'd break loose and be harder to control. From the age of five years old, I remember mustering cattle.

I was gifted my first stockwhip by the time I was seven. I started riding not much after that. Even though I wasn't much bigger than a grasshopper to these much larger beasts, they would avoid me, even when I was on foot. To them, I was a predator. They were afraid of me. It was in their DNA. Lucky for me, they were scared.

Early on, when you start mustering, you get a feel for what the cattle will do. If they begin to wander to the side rather than go straight ahead, you'd soon see their change of focus. Then you'd go wide so they could see you in the corner of their eye, and most of the time, they'd straighten up again. The cattle were reactive. This reactive nature helped us muster, corral, tag, inject and castrate them, and send them in trucks to markets or the abattoir. But what if they were less reactive and more strategic?

Imagine trying to round up a herd of cattle that knew they would be tortured or killed. Imagine if cattle weren't so easily controlled using fear. There is no way they would let a short snotty-nosed kid in jeans, checked shirt and gumboots with a noise-maker push them around. It'd take enormous force to get them to do anything. They wouldn't be so easily led.

We have learned many insights about the nature of fear and how to tame it. Among the wisdom, we have learned how fear can bother us when we don't want it to, such as worrying about work when at home with the family, or so dominate our minds that we struggle to switch it off without conscious will. Fear can make it next to impossible to not think of worst cases, such as having a severe illness or something terrible happening. Fear can even make us do what we intuitively know we shouldn't, such as becoming scared of others to the point of isolation, being quick to blame or being angry with those we love and in so doing ruin our relationships. And, to top it off, fear can make us so busy we are bouncing like a pinball from one activity to another, without time to scratch, let alone reflect and contemplate. Whether they are Covid-related or not, our fears can take control of our lives.

My internal journey in my early twenties taught me many invaluable insights about fear. Some I have shared with you so that you too can tame fear in your life. But once we know the truth of fear's nature, one final and crucial realisation stares us in the face: fear can corral us like cattle.

This concerning revelation shouldn't come as a big surprise. We have already learned how our brains can be easily led when dominated by fear.

When we discovered fear's great secret, we learned that our brain shuts off planning and rational problem solving and demands we react when we are afraid. This ability to be stronger, faster and think more quickly in the moment can be lifesaving. It can be particularly advantageous if we don't know what to do – if we have no memory to fall back on. But this ability becomes our Achilles heel.

For all the lifesaving qualities of fear, it is also primarily toxic.

Unless we walk with fear and talk to it regularly, it can lead us down dangerous paths that we may not know we are taking until it is too late. Untamed fear doesn't just cage us and restrict our lives; it spurs us to run our path blindly until we can't stop, even when at the edge of the cliff. Fear prevents us from being strategic.

In other words, the more we stay in an uncontrolled fear-like state, the more we become reactive like cattle.

It's easy to find ourselves in this predicament, isn't it? We don't have many supports. We do the job of two or three people, come home, clean, cook, do the books and study. We catch up with others if we have the time. We are scared every day by what we read or see. We avoid taming our fears. We let them loose. We let them lead us. We react.

Kallie, Carol and Melinda were classic examples of people so pushed by anxiety they don't spend time planning or contemplating; they just react. They barely see more than a few steps into the future. How many of us are like Kallie, Carol and Melinda in the rushed modern lifestyle of today? How many of us are being corralled like cattle?

And while we are being corralled, we are being robbed of choice. Let fear run rampant in the background or foreground of our lives, and we take away full, conscious choice.

That is what being strategic is: it is choosing – choosing how we live, how we feel and how we act, knowing how it will affect us and those around us in the future.

How have your fears robbed you of your potential? Have you felt you have been guiding your life or that your fears have been controlling it for you, corralling you into the yards or the truck they want?

I could have mentioned in the introduction how fear robs us of choice. But then, you may not have fully appreciated what fear stealing us of choice meant, not until you tamed your fear and could look back.

The more I have explored fear in all its forms and variations, the more it has taught me a great lesson. We should keep fear as low as possible as much as possible personally, especially socially.

Imagine a life where we weren't scared of others. Instead, we took the time to know them and contemplate their way of seeing things. How much better would we get along?

With less fear, would we have so many conflicts? So many wars?

What if we made reducing fear in our society a top priority? How might our communities change? Would we check on each other more? Would genuine care be restored to neighbourhoods and suburbs?

Taming fear in the age of Covid is more than reducing a fear burden or taming a nagging fear that has bothered us. It is more than rewriting the fear of trauma from childhood or domestic violence. What if taming fear is also a positive act of empowerment, a restoration of choice? What if us taming fear is our act of saving ourselves from being led like cattle to slaughter?

The more I understand the nature of fear, the more I see hope for us. We live in challenging times. Covid and looming or current wars have stressed us. But the fears they trigger are a great opportunity. We can finally learn to walk in peace, hand in hand, calmly, with our new friend: tamed fear. And as the fog of fear settles, we are in a much better position to choose our future rather than have it dictated to us.

What kind of world would you choose to live in if you could?

How would you like to feel in that world? How would you like our children to feel?

Have you made taming fear a priority in your life?

APPENDIX 1: THE BALANCE OF SELF MODEL

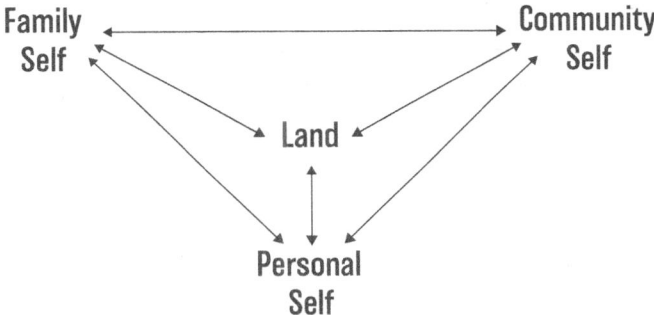

The components explained

Personal Self

Personal Self represents the desires and motivations that allow us to survive as individuals in our own right, without others; for example, the desires to satisfy our hunger and thirst and our need for shelter.

Personal Self can also be considered to have five defining qualities:

1. self-worth
2. self-respect
3. being your best friend
4. our personal unique connection with the world
5. sense of choice.

Family Self

Family Self represents the desires and motivations that drive us to be part of families and have our own families. These desires change as we mature. The Family Self desires of a child will be different from those of an adult.

Community Self

Community Self represents the desires for us to form and be part of a supportive social group – a community or tribe. We can distinguish ten basic desires of Community Self we all seek to have satisfied. We all strive to feel:

1. valued
2. noticed
3. appreciated
4. heard
5. sameness
6. validated/approved
7. respected
8. cared for
9. supported
10. protected.

These same ten desires can also be regarded as ten desires of friendship. They have been briefly described earlier in Chapter 7.

Land

Land represents everything that is not human. Essentially it represents nature and the natural world.

Coexistence and the Balance of Components

You will notice all the components have arrows connected to the other parts. This indicates that none of these components exist independently and that each is influenced by the others. For instance, our level of Personal Self will be determined by how valued it is by family and community. If families and communities do not value, or respect, a strong sense of Personal Self, we can expect to struggle to develop a sound and genuine sense of self and identity. Similarly, Land – nature – affects all other components. For example, the land we live on will determine our family sizes according to available resources and our culture, which is an integral part of our sense of community. Likewise, Land determines the nature of our language, art, technology and culinary cuisine.

The Balance of Self Model reminds us of the essential balance we need between time for self, family, community and Land – Country. It reminds us how we must balance our humanity's fundamentals and basic human needs. For example, to spend too much time at work – Community Self – compared to our individual and family needs indicates self-imbalance. The greater the imbalance and expected future imbalance, the less satisfied we feel.

* * * * *

For further detail see my book *A Balance of Self: A New Approach to Self-Understanding, Lasting Happiness, and Self-Truth* (Vivid Publishing, Fremantle, 2011).

ACKNOWLEDGEMENTS

The privilege I have experienced helping clients has always been a two-way street. Mutual learning has been at the core of helping others find release from mental illness. This book would not have been possible were it not for the patience and courage of amazing people placing their trust in our collaboration. So, first, and with profound appreciation, I humbly thank everyone I have had the honour to know and treat over the decades, especially the last ten years. You all played a crucial part.

Next, I would like to offer a big thank you to my editor, Susan Lee. I appreciate her professionalism, feedback, and especially the personal real-life anecdotes she kindly shared. The book is clearer and easier to read, thanks to Susan.

Another big thank you goes to the book's graphic designer, George Stevens. Our collaboration has been a delight and enormously fruitful. The cover wouldn't be so striking and the text not so well laid out were it not for George.

Thank you to my mental health supervision group colleagues for your ongoing support, feedback, shared wisdom, and valued experience. Our twice-monthly meetings are always a highlight.

Finally, thank you to family, friends and the many people who helped shape my life over the years. This book is a culmination of a lifetime. Every experience with others over my existence is needed to make it what it is.

www.ingramcontent.com/pod-product-compliance
Lightning Source LLC
Chambersburg PA
CBHW070530010526
44118CB00012B/1092